T0174429

The Age of Ageing Better?

The Age of Ageing Better?

A MANIFESTO FOR OUR FUTURE

Dr Anna Dixon

GREEN TREE
LONDON • OXFORD • NEW YORK • NEW DELHI • SYDNEY

Dedicated to my parents and grandparents

GREEN TREE
Bloomsbury Publishing Plc
50 Bedford Square, London, WC1B 3DP, UK

BLOOMSBURY, GREEN TREE and the Green Tree logo are trademarks of
Bloomsbury Publishing Plc

First published in Great Britain 2020

Copyright © Anna Dixon, 2020

Illustrations by David Gardner, 2020

Anna Dixon has asserted her right under the Copyright, Designs and
Patents Act, 1988, to be identified as Author of this work

For legal purposes the Acknowledgements on p. 290 constitute
an extension of this copyright page

All rights reserved. No part of this publication may be reproduced or transmitted in
any form or by any means, electronic or mechanical, including photocopying,
recording, or any information storage or retrieval system, without prior
permission in writing from the publishers

Bloomsbury Publishing Plc does not have any control over, or responsibility for,
any third-party websites referred to or in this book. All Internet addresses given
in this book were correct at the time of going to press. The author and publisher
regret any inconvenience caused if addresses have changed or sites have ceased
to exist, but can accept no responsibility for any such changes

A catalogue record for this book is available from the British Library

Library of Congress Cataloguing-in-Publication data has been applied for

ISBN: TPB: 978-1-4729-6073-3; eBook: 978-1-4729-6072-6

2 4 6 8 10 9 7 5 3

Typeset in Sabon by Deanta Global Publishing Services, Chennai, India
Printed and bound in Great Britain by CPI Group (UK) Ltd, Croydon CR0 4YY

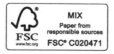

To find out more about our authors and books visit www.bloomsbury.com
and sign up for our newsletters

Contents

Foreword

I am writing this preface in April 2020. These are strange and worrying times. It is older people, especially with other conditions, who are most at risk of serious illness or death resulting from infection by the Covid 19 virus. Ever since the crisis began there have been those who have explicitly or by insinuation asked why society should be locked down and the economy crashed to save people 'who would have died soon anyway'. Once again, we have been reminded of how much we rely on the caring professions and how negligent of them we are in normal times.

The vulnerability of some older people, the prevalence of ageism, our inadequate approach to care; these are all among the themes addressed by Anna Dixon in this authoritative, wide-ranging and cogent analysis of our current approach to an ageing society and what needs to change. Within these pages we can also read about work, housing, pensions and even loneliness. In contrast to the popular myth, Dixon points out that loneliness is less prevalent among the old than the young.

This observation is typical of a book which is motivated by a passionate commitment to getting ageing right for society and individuals, but which avoids being emotive or rhetorical, focusing instead on the facts and on practical solutions ranging from Government strategy to lifestyle decisions.

I share with Anna Dixon a view of change that we can and we should combine big visions and ideals with pragmatic, multi-faceted solutions. This book will help you as a campaigner for age equality, as an advocate for better policy but also as a responsible employer or simply as a good citizen.

I reach my own seventh decade later this year. My gratitude to Anna Dixon for producing this excellent rejoinder to lazy pessimism about an ageing society is not just professional but personal.

Matthew Taylor,
Chief Executive of the Royal Society
for the Encouragement of Arts

Introducing the Age of Ageing Better

Do you ever wonder what the world will be like when you get old? You probably don't consider yourself old now – few people do. And what about your children or your grandchildren? What will their old age be like?

I don't know about you, but when I think about my future, I want to be active and independent. I want to stay in the community where I now live (no retiring to the seaside for me!), to be able to get around easily, to meet up with my friends, go to the cinema and theatre, simply to carry on with the many things I enjoy now. I want to live my life to the full, to the very end.

So why is it when we hear the term 'ageing society' we imagine care homes full of people with dementia sitting around staring at the TV screen, hospitals full to overflowing with patients (or 'bed blockers'), lonely 80-somethings trapped in their own homes? We hear so often about the problems of an ageing society that it can distance us from the issue, when, in fact, ageing is deeply personal and impacts on absolutely everyone – you, your friends, your family. It is universal and it is global.

Few of us think of ourselves as old, whether we're 60, 70 or 80. A recent YouGov survey found that it was only in the 70-and-above age bracket that a majority of respondents described themselves as old (59%). Only a third of those aged 65-69 did (35%), and less than a fifth of those aged 60-64 (19%).[1] And yet all of us are ageing. Ageing is a natural biological process. It starts when we are about 30. For some, such as those who are exposed to heavy loads of environmental stressors like pollution, smoking and alcohol, as well as psychological stress, it happens more quickly. Others remain biologically 'young' for longer, remaining fit and healthy into their 90s. Chronological age, as you will come to understand from reading this book, doesn't indicate very much at all about us.

Is there an age at which old age starts? The age at which people perceive 'old age' begins varies by country. It is a culturally-relative concept. While a majority of British people think that a person of 59 is old, in Greece most people believe old age starts at 68.[2] It also depends on the context. For example, when we talk about older workers, we often mean those over 50, but different studies use different age cut-offs, depending on the data available. Lots of studies use 65, as this has been the state pension age for men for a long time, although it is now rising. Because of inequalities in how long we can expect to live, later life could be said to start 15 years earlier for someone living in a poor area than for someone in a rich area. And given how quickly life expectancy has risen in every generation, old age for today's 30-year-olds may well start later than it did for someone who is 70 today.

Thanks to advances in medical science, improvements in public health and rising living standards, many diseases which would have led to death or disability in the past, are now preventable or survivable. We are living longer than ever before – longevity is the new reality.

As more of us survive longer and the birth rate remains low, the proportion of 'old' to 'young' is changing and it's changing fast. More of us are older than ever before in history. For the first time ever in the UK, there are more people aged 60 and over than there are aged 19 and below. This has been true in Europe since 2005, but globally it is not predicted to be the case until 2080.[3] This change in the demographic composition of the population is often referred to as the 'ageing population' or 'ageing society'. I prefer to call this demographic change the 'age shift'.

The age shift is a global issue. Some countries have already experienced this dramatic change in the age profile of the population and in a more extreme way than the UK. For example, in Japan, people are living longer than in the UK, and birth rates and levels of immigration, which traditionally brings in younger age groups, are lower. But there are also rapidly industrialising countries that are following hot on our heels and will experience these changes even more swiftly than developed countries have. For example, improvements in health and living standards, at least for the emerging middle classes, in countries like Brazil mean that the share of the population over 65 is predicted to increase from 7% to 14% in just two decades, the same demographic transition which took a hundred years to happen in France.[4]

These profound changes are already changing the way we live today, impacting on many aspects of our lives, from our finances and our health to our workplaces and our homes. And they are set to radically change how we live in the future. Many people predict these changes will have negative impacts, bankrupting public finances, overwhelming our health and care services, taking jobs from young people and denying them the chance to own their own homes. I call these naysayers 'the doom-mongers'. They come in many guises – economists, politicians, journalists, commentators and, yes, academics. While some of the impacts of this age shift are challenging – I won't pretend otherwise when the evidence and data show this – it is not all doom and gloom. Some of the predictions are over-hyped or misinterpret the facts. Other potential consequences of the age shift can be averted if we take action now. And yet society is failing to respond with the urgency required.

We're all guilty of failing to fully comprehend what this means for our families, for our businesses and for our communities, but why? Why do we all have our heads so firmly buried in the sand?

Maybe it's because we're afraid of getting old. Or because we're paralysed by the size and scale of the challenge. Or because we are distracted by immediate economic and political concerns. Perhaps it seems less pressing than some of the other major challenges we face. I want to convince you that we should be tackling this issue with the same urgency as global issues like climate change.

We face a choice: carry on as if nothing is happening or respond to this social revolution now. How we react will shape the future, a future in which more people experience ill health and disability for longer, live in poverty and worry about money, and feel excluded from society, or one in which the growing numbers of people in later life are happy, healthy, financially secure and able to contribute fully to society. How can we ensure that we live in the age of ageing better and not in the age of ageing badly? In this book I'll put forward and analyse some of the radical solutions which could help us turn the challenge into an opportunity.

While the age shift is a global phenomenon, this book focuses on solutions for the UK context. Devolution means there are significant differences in some policy areas, such as health, between the countries of the UK. Where this is the case I focus on England. I take ideas from other countries, but context matters and solutions that work in one place or country often don't work somewhere else. We don't start with a blank canvas. The institutions that exist create particular ways of doing things. Our culture and beliefs shape our attitudes and actions, and our economic and political situation makes some changes easier and others harder. Timing also matters: the economic cycle, elections and political events shape opportunities or put up barriers.

I started my career working for the World Health Organisation, supporting health policy makers in Eastern Europe and the former Soviet Union to reform their health systems. Most of the research and policy ideas came from Western Europe, where they had been implemented in the context of economic growth, political stability and by long-established institutions like the NHS in the UK or sickness funds in Germany. I learnt quickly that adaptation rather than adoption was needed. As well as this book being deeply relevant to the future of the UK, I hope readers from other countries will find the ideas here of interest and be able to take and adapt them to their situation.

The scale of the changes we face means there's an urgent need to prepare for them and respond to them. Many aspects of our society are impacted by this age shift in the population. It has implications for the welfare state, for financial services, for health and social care services, for housing, for employers, for voluntary and community services, for education and training, for planning and transport, for relationships and family life. There are implications for every facet of our lives. We need to radically change the places where we work, live and play.

There is much we can and need to do as individuals. Through youth and middle age, we need to think about the pattern of our working lives, including the potential to work for longer, retrain or work more flexibly. We need to manage our finances throughout life with a realistic view about how long we might live. And, of course, try to stay healthy and fit, find time for friends, think about where we'll live, and how we'll keep active and make a contribution. If you want to know more about what you personally can do to have a great later life, then I'd recommend *When We're 64: Your Guide to a Great Later Life*, written by my colleague at the Centre for Ageing Better, Louise Ansari.

This book is for those of you who believe in society; who as citizens want everyone to enjoy a good later life; who want to make a difference not only for your own future, but for that of generations to come. In each chapter I'll assess the current situation, challenging some of the arguments put forward, and reviewing the evidence and facts. I'll consider the implications if we carry on as we are and make the case for change. I'll look at some of the solutions available to us and how different things could be if we had the courage to act. However, I am not naïve enough to imagine that all the changes I advocate in this book can be implemented easily, because some require bold economic and political decisions.

My motivation in writing this book is to make a difference in the world. I have a privileged position as Chief Executive of the Centre for Ageing Better. I have access to so much rich knowledge and insights that I can share with you. There is no point in only me knowing what employers need to do to enable more people to work for longer. On my own I can only do something for the 50-odd people who work in my organisation, but each one of you can make a difference where you work.

I can help my parents think about moving to a more suitable house and support my mother-in-law to adapt her home, but if you're involved in architecture, design, retail, construction, home building, housing associations or planning, you can reshape the homes that we all live in. I can talk to friends, my husband and wider family, people in my church, my colleagues and others in my personal and social spheres about the importance of planning ahead, but these kinds of conversations are important for all of us. These issues need wider exposure to achieve greater impact.

In this book I draw on a wide range of sources, including:

The latest published research and evidence: For the past four years I have led a new organisation called the Centre for Ageing Better. We have been pulling together existing research and have also commissioned new research, including a major study with Ipsos Mori of the experiences of people over 50, which I draw on throughout the book. I refer to it as the Later Life Study. I'll introduce you to the six groups we identified in this research in a moment, as these 'types' or 'segments' recur throughout the book.

Case studies and innovative examples: through our work we try to identify practical examples of where potentially exciting new approaches are being tried out. We support a network of age-friendly communities across the UK and work in partnership with other local areas. This gives us unique insight into what is happening on the ground. The issues we are dealing with are global and many other countries are trying to find solutions, too. The book also includes some international examples.

Expert opinion: my role has also given me privileged access to some of the leading experts in their fields who generously gave time to be interviewed for this book. In places I have directly quoted them or paraphrased our conversations. However, their insights and ideas contributed richly to my own thinking, for which I am grateful.

Facts and data: thankfully for those of us who like facts and numbers, this area is rich in data. The Office for National Statistics in the UK has taken a leading role to ensure major public data sources are broken down by age so we can look at the differences between different age groups. The other major dataset that many of the research studies use, which I cite directly and which also formed the basis for the Later Life Study I mentioned earlier, is the English Longitudinal Study of Ageing (ELSA). This is a cohort study, which means the researchers go back and ask questions of the same people each time. The survey started in 2002 and has been repeated seven times, the most recent one being in 2018. It covers health, work, finances, homes and wellbeing, among other things.

Personal stories and experiences: I have included some personal stories from my own life as well as some from people we have spoken to in the course of our work at the Centre for Ageing Better. In this book I have written about issues which will affect me, my family, friends and work colleagues, the people on my street and in my social circles. In fact, I can think of individuals where specific issues related to health or work, for example, will really hit hard if we don't change our systems and structures. I'm sure this will be the same for you, and your friends and family.

I will lay out a vision for how our society could be different; a vision of a society where we are all able to make the most of our longer lives, where old age is celebrated not feared, and where people of all ages and abilities feel part of their communities. I believe such a vision can become reality. In the final chapter, I set out how that can happen.

1

The changing face of the population

'It's more about how we live than about how long we live.'
Jo Ann Jenkins, CEO of AARP[1]

Most books on ageing start with statistics about how many old people there will be in future. What they fail to convey is that this is about you and me. It's about us. On average, we will live 10 years longer than our parents' generation and 20 years longer than our grandparents' generation. This is not some future issue only of concern to strategists and futurologists. This is happening now. This is a story about every generation alive today. So, what is the true scale of this age shift we are living through?

There are two main drivers of the dramatic shift in the age profile of the population. First, longevity, the fact that on average we are living longer than previous generations. Second, people born during the post-war and 1960s baby booms are reaching later life: the first group, born shortly after World War II (1946-49), have already celebrated their 65th birthdays and the second group, born in the 1960s, are in their 50s in 2019 and are fast approaching later life. Let's look at the first of these factors: longevity and the changes in life span.

LONGER LIVES

We are living longer than ever before. A lot longer. The change in life expectancy over the last century is truly staggering. A baby boy born in 1916 in England could have expected to live to about 58. A baby boy born in 2016 can expect to see his 90th birthday.[2] You could call it a 'megatrend' created by shared human endeavour, because advances in public health, science and medicine, and improved living standards, have caused a social revolution.

These improvements have continued apace over the past 20 years. Men's life expectancy at birth increased from 75 to 79 between 1998 and 2017 (a 6% increase) and life expectancy at 65 increased from 15.4 years to 19 years over the same time period (a 20% increase).[3] According to the Office of National Statistics, the commonest age of death in 2015-2017 was 83 for women and 79 for men. These figures represent more than four extra years for men since 2001-2003, and nearly three more years for women.[4] This is a remarkable and profound change.

While in the past, gains in life expectancy were due to actions to avoid premature death, such as improvements in sanitation, the advent of antibiotics, mass childhood immunisation and improvements in childhood nutrition and hygiene, in recent years it's been because of extending life at older ages, particularly among men – effectively we have postponed death.[5]

THE CHANGING PATTERN OF MORTALITY

Many of these increases have been due to the narrowing of the gender gap between men and women's life expectancy, which has been attributed, at least in part, to a reduction in the number of men smoking at older ages and the prevention of death from heart disease through more effective, widespread use of statins (drugs taken to lower cholesterol).[6] Improvements in detection and treatment of cancer have also resulted in extended life expectancy. Although there are differences by gender and income, in 2015 cancer was still the most common cause of death (28% of all deaths registered), followed by circulatory diseases, such as heart disease and strokes (26%).[7]

While public health measures and improved medical treatment mean we have combatted some of the causes of premature death, we are still dying from other diseases, albeit at older ages. In the past it was acceptable for a doctor to simply say someone had died of old age or 'senility', although this has no real medical definition. In 2014 just 7,500 people in the UK died of 'senility'.[8] Generally, over the last decade, causes of death have been more accurately recorded. Reforms to death certification to improve their accuracy and introduce safeguards were implemented in 2007 as a response to the Inquiry into the GP Harold Shipman, who murdered 250 mostly elderly patients.[9]

As deaths from other causes have declined, dementia has become a more common cause of death. Overall, death certificates with dementia or Alzheimer's as the underlying cause rose from 13,200 in 2006 (3% of all deaths) to 67,641 in 2017 (13% of all deaths).[10] This is partly because diagnosis of dementia is improving. GPs receive some funding to accurately diagnose and monitor long-term conditions, including dementia, and to monitor and review care plans for these patients.[11] As people living to very old ages survive other diseases, we can expect the numbers of people dying from (or with?) dementia to continue to increase. Among those over 90, nearly 30% have dementia and more than 40% of people over 95 years old have it.[12]

There are worrying trends that these amazing increases in our life span, driven by falling mortality at older ages from the big killers – heart disease, stroke and cancer – are about to come to an end, particularly for people living in the most deprived areas.

ARE THE GAINS IN LIFE EXPECTANCY COMING TO AN END?

Life expectancy growth has levelled off since 2011, as has the reduction in mortality rates. This sounds pretty bad news, doesn't it? What's happening and why? Such has been the concern in government that Public Health England (PHE), a government agency responsible for protecting and improving the health of the population, was asked to undertake further analysis of the changes and the reasons for the slowdown. There are a number of different ways to measure life expectancy and, by all such measures, life expectancy increases are slowing.

Official statistics most commonly use what is called 'period life expectancy' for projections, although this tends to underestimate life expectancy increases in the future, because it assumes that the mortality rates at a particular age today will not change in the future. An alternative method called 'cohort life expectancy' makes a set of assumptions which influence how mortality rates for different cohorts (people born in the same year) are calculated. For example, it might assume that advances in medical technology will mean that mortality rates for cancer or heart disease will be lower in the future than they are today or perhaps that rates of smoking among younger generations will mean lower mortality rates from smoking-related diseases. The common measure of life span for both period and cohort is life expectancy at birth. However, more relevant for understanding longevity is to look at life expectancy at age 65, since this gives us a better idea of how many people can expect to live to the oldest ages.

There had been sustained improvements in all measures of life expectancy for the majority of the 20th century and the beginning of the 21st century. If we first look at life expectancy at birth, we can see that life expectancy for women at birth increased by one year every five years. For example, a baby girl born in 2001-2003 had a life expectancy of 80.5 at birth. A baby girl born a few years later, in 2005-2007 had a life expectancy of 81.5. However, the steady gains in life expectancy have all but disappeared in the latest period. If we look a decade later, a girl born in 2011-13 had a life expectancy of 82.8 and one born in 2015-17 had an almost identical life expectancy of 82.9 at birth.[13]

The professor behind much of this research, Sir Michael Marmot, Director of University College London's Institute of Health Equity, said this was 'historically highly unusual' and expressed deep concern at the fact that life expectancy growth is 'pretty close to having ground to a halt' when he had expected it to get better. While a similar slowdown was found in other European Union countries, the UK had the slowest rate of improvement.[14]

The 2018 Public Health England report, *Review of recent trends in mortality in England*, found that gains in life expectancy had slowed most in the most deprived areas of the country: for some groups in some parts of England increases in life expectancy had stopped altogether and for women in the most deprived areas life expectancy had actually gone backwards. For women in the poorest tenth of the population, life expectancy at birth in 2011-2013 was 79.0; by 2015-2017 this had dropped slightly to 78.7. Meanwhile, over the same period, the life expectancy at birth for women in the wealthiest tenth of the population had increased from 85.9 to 86.2. Similarly, life expectancy at age 65 for women in the poorest tenth fell from 18.6 to 18.4 years, while for women in the wealthiest tenth of the population it increased from 22.9 to 23.2 years.[15] It seems the slowdown in life expectancy is hitting the poorest hardest.

Various reasons for this have been mooted, including that the recession, austerity, job quality and security, and growing income inequalities may be having an impact. Academics in the US have analysed trends in mortality rates there to try and understand the factors causing a rise in mortality rates at younger ages in America (see box on the next page).

The Public Health England report doesn't point to a single issue and certainly doesn't lay the blame solely with austerity, although writing in the BMJ's blog, Veena Raleigh, senior fellow at the King's Fund, an independent health charity, commented that, 'It's possible that public expenditure cuts accelerated or even precipitated some deaths, especially among frail, older people.' [16]

Deaths during winter, particularly of sicker and frailer people and those with dementia, and a bad flu outbreak in 2015, partly skew the figures. Doing more to ensure people are vaccinated against flu and have adequate heating and insulation in their homes would help. As we will see in the chapter on housing, local authorities no longer have funding to provide loans to low income owner-occupiers to improve the heating and insulation of their homes, so austerity is partly to blame. And the significant gains that have been made historically in preventing deaths from heart

LEARNING FROM THE DEATHS OF DESPAIR IN AMERICA

Professors Anne Case and Angus Deaton, prominent professors of economics, found that the decline in life expectancy among white non-Hispanic Americans with fewer qualifications is a result of increases in what they call 'deaths of despair' – that is suicide, and mortality from liver disease due to alcohol and drug overdoses. These are seen most dramatically among those in mid-life.[17] Deaton and Case argue that the increasing rates of mortality among younger birth cohorts are the result of 'cumulative disadvantage' including falling real wages and living standards, higher skill roles being replaced by insecure and poor-quality jobs, and the loss of family and household support networks, which in turn undermine status and leave people with little meaning and purpose (a key driver of wellbeing). Deaton plans to conduct a similar analysis of the situation in the UK.

We have a stronger safety net in the UK than in the US, mostly in the form of unemployment benefits, but this doesn't necessarily substitute for the benefits of 'good' work. It seems the US pattern of deaths of despair is different to other countries which have had greater economic liberalisation, including the UK, Canada, Australia, France, Germany and Sweden. It remains to be seen whether other countries will follow the US pattern in the future as changes in the availability and nature of work impact on those with low education and skills or whether differences in economic and labour market policies will mitigate the effects.

disease and stroke are slowing down, suggesting a need to step up efforts to prevent these by tackling smoking, high blood pressure and obesity, which are particular problems among lower socio-economic groups. However, it's important to note that increases in death rates were seen in all age groups, not just the older ones.

Looking ahead, there is also concern about the impact of obesity and related diseases on future life expectancy, although the links between obesity and mortality have weakened slightly due to improvements in treatment and improved survival from cardiovascular disease since the 1970s.[18] Higher levels of obesity are also likely to have significant adverse effects on quality of life, with longer periods spent with disability in later life.

The slow-down in gains in life expectancy and increasing mortality rates from diseases that should be preventable and other causes at younger ages is a worrying trend. These growing social and economic inequalities risk reversing some of the gains in life expectancy for the poorest and most disadvantaged in our society. Nonetheless, the prospect of a longer life span than previous generations is a reality for many of us. But how long can we expect to live?

IS THERE AN UPPER LIMIT TO OUR HUMAN LIFESPAN?

Do you know someone who is 100? According to the Office of National Statistics there were 3,000 centenarians in 1983. This rose to 14,500 in 2016.[19] The number of centenarians worldwide has also increased exponentially in the last three decades. At least 434,000 people were thought to have reached their 100th birthday in 2015, compared to 90,000 in 1990. While the global population increased by more than a third (38%) between 1990 and 2015, the number of centenarians rose by nearly 400% (382%).[20]

We still find these people amazing, don't we? This is perhaps not so surprising given that someone born in 1914 had just a 1% chance of reaching 100.[21] Now think of a child you know under the age of 10. That child has more than a 50% chance of living to 100.[22] There are differences between countries, though, so while in the UK half of the babies born in 2007 are predicted to still be alive at age 103, in Japan half of the babies born that year are expected to live to 107.[23]

Some scientists and a number of high-profile individuals, mainly American men with fortunes made in Silicon Valley, don't believe we have reached the limits yet of the human life span and are investing personally and professionally in pushing the limits of longevity.[24]

Epidemiologists such as James Fries, writing in the 1980s, argued that there is a finite life span; that even if we could prevent all disease, natural death would occur for everyone in a particular cohort before a certain age. This is called the 'maximum life potential' and was estimated by the oldest age of any human; which was just over 113 years old in the US at the time.[25] The oldest person thought to have ever lived, Jeanne Calment, died age 122 in 1997. This suggests that there is still quite a long way to go before we reach the limits of longevity.

DO WE KNOW HOW LONG WE WILL LIVE?

I discovered recently that I have a 50% chance of living to 93. This came as a bit of a shock. Given my job you might have thought I would have known this already and yet for some reason it hadn't sunk in. It was only when I got a personalised prediction from one of the online life expectancy calculators that I exclaimed 'OMG!'

And I'm not alone. Many of us underestimate how long we will live. Perhaps we focus on those we know, our parents and grandparents, and use the age at which they died as a guide to how long we might live. Or perhaps it's because the changes have been so rapid, our perceptions have not kept up with reality. Research by the Institute for Fiscal Studies (IFS), a leading economics research institute, found that on average our expectations of how long we will live are about a fifth lower than the estimates of survival using data. It also found that the least wealthy, those with lower levels of formal education and people who are widowed, were more pessimistic (i.e. there was a bigger gap between their expectations and estimates).[26]

Why does this matter? For a start we might not save enough for retirement or spend down our pension savings too quickly. It might also mean we engage less with preventative health checks or fail to seek medical help if we think we have less time to live than we actually do. We might stop paid work earlier than we should or put up with a home that's not suitable for our needs rather than planning ahead.

The fact that we are living longer is just one of the factors driving the dramatic age shift we are seeing in the population. We now turn to the other factor that makes the changes to the age profile of our population so dramatic – the 'baby boomers' of the early 1960s are approaching later life.

THE BABY BOOM BULGE REACHES OLD AGE

The proportion of old to young in this country is changing and it's changing fast. In 2000, there were 9.3 million people over 65.[27] By 2019 the number of people over 65 had grown to 12 million[28] and estimates suggest that by 2039 we can expect to see a staggering 18 million people over 65.[29] This surge in the number of older people is in large part due to the baby boomers reaching old age.

While the number of live births in the UK fluctuated during the 20th century (see graph on page 18), there were two peaks after each of the World Wars. Although more babies were born after the end of World War I (957,782 in 1920) than at the end of World War II (820,719 in 1946), many more of those in the latter group have survived to older ages, so 78% of babies born in 1946 turned 70 years old in 2016, whereas only 58% of those born in 1920 lived long enough to see their 70th birthday in 1990.[30] There was also a longer 'boom' during the 1960s, and in every year between 1961 and 1968 inclusive, the number of births per year exceeded 800,000.[31]

In most analyses, the baby boomers are defined as those born between 1945 and 1965. These lump together the post-World War II boom and the early part of the 1960s boom to create a single generation, but this includes a dip in the 1950s. This definition of the baby boomers is closer to the pattern of births in the US, which grew steadily after the war and remained at a peak between 1957 and 1961. The group I am particularly interested in is the UK baby boomers of the 1960s, who are currently in their 50s (I will always indicate which definition of baby boomer a study refers to). Between 1960 and 1969 inclusive there were over 8.3 million births in the UK.[32] This age shift is only just getting started in the UK and will be with us for the next two or three decades. It will not be until around 2050 that the 1960s baby boomer cohort reaches the oldest ages and begins to die off.

The later baby boomers differ in significant ways from the post-World War II boomers who are now in their early to mid-70s. For example, their pension benefits are not as good. While many of the 1960s baby boomers had access to a defined benefit pension (one that guarantees a certain income linked to your salary) in their early working lives, many of these schemes closed and switched to defined contribution pensions (where the amount you have on retirement depends on the amount of savings and how investments have performed) in the latter part of their working lives. Many of this generation are

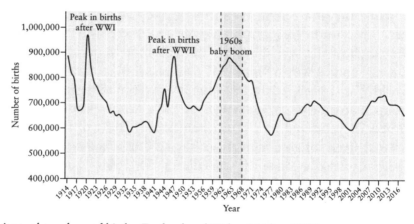

Annual numbers of births, England and Wales, 1914 to 2018.

Source: Office of National Statistics (2019), Births in England and Wales: summary tables, 2018-based.

homeowners – more than half of those born in the 1960s were homeowners by the age of 26[33] – and while house prices and interest rates were higher than for the previous generation, they have enjoyed huge increases in property values. Social housing tenants also benefitted from Right to Buy, introduced under Margaret Thatcher in 1980, which allowed them to purchase the property they rented at a substantially discounted rate. As we explore the issues in more detail in later chapters, we'll consider how these differences might impact on the experience of later life and what some of the solutions might be to reduce any potential negative consequences for society.

The sheer numbers and the fact that they are about to reach their 60s means the 1960s baby boomers will drive the dramatic age shift over the next 20 to 30 years, but the predictions that the age shift will bring dire consequences need not necessarily come true. It is not inevitable that these people will experience the same challenges faced by some of today's older generation. If we act now, we have the chance to respond to this age shift and change the experience of later life for generations to come.

THE CHANGING AGE PROFILE OF THE POPULATION

So far, we have looked at the dramatic increases in life span and the fact that the baby boomers of the 1960s are entering later life. The age shift in the population is also affected by the birth rate and by migration. As the example of Japan shows (see box on page 20), it is not only longevity but also a falling birth rate and low levels of immigration that cause an age shift towards more older people.[34] The birth rate in the UK fell during the 1990s, increased steadily between 2002 and 2012, and has declined slightly again in recent years. Relative to the baby boomers these subsequent cohorts are much smaller. Tighter immigration controls and the UK's departure from the European Union will make increasing the population through migration less likely.

JAPAN – ONE OF THE OLDEST COUNTRIES ON EARTH

Japan has the second-highest median age in the world, after Monaco. Half of its residents are younger than 48 and half older, and more than 20% of its population are over 70.[35] Japan's rapid age shift has largely been due to population longevity and very low fertility rates. The dwindling population is probably best illustrated by the fact that there were 8.2 million more homes than there were households to fill them in 2013, so some local areas were giving away homes for free.[36]

Fertility rates have been below replacement level since the early 1970s. This means that there are more deaths than births and the people who die are not 'replaced', so the population shrinks as a result. Japan's population of 127.4 million people in 2017 is expected to reduce to 108.7 million by 2050.[37] Despite 40 years of low marriage and fertility rates, the government has been slow to react. Actions to encourage marriage and reduce gender inequality in family life and the workplace were not set in motion until the 1990s. Recent legislation has concentrated on making Japan more family-friendly, for example, with the recent introduction of free childcare for pre-school age children.

Historically reluctant to recruit immigrant workers, there has been a slow acceptance of the need to boost the working population, but there is little political desire for workers to settle permanently. Although there will be more than a quarter of a million visas available to unskilled guest workers from 2019, these are only of five years' duration. Instead, the government has attempted to get more people into work and for them to work longer. This is particularly important in a country where about 60% of women leave paid employment for at least a decade after the birth of their first child.[38]

While Japan is often looked to as a country to learn from, in fact other countries have also recognised the age shift as a major strategic issue that requires a cross-government and cross-sectoral response. Australia published a national strategy in 2001. In the foreword the then Prime Minister of Australia, John Howard, wrote, 'The ageing of the Australian population is something that will touch all facets of our personal and community lives. The challenges flowing from this inevitable demographic change will have significant implications for all sectors of our nation.'[39] New Zealand also published a *Positive Ageing Strategy* in 2001, recognising the positive contribution that older people make to society.[40] Singapore also has embraced the age shift as a positive opportunity and has set out its ambitions in a plan for what is called 'successful ageing' (see box on page 22).

A common way of presenting the age profile of the population is by calculating the so-called old age dependency ratio (OADR). This gives the ratio of the number of people over a certain age (usually 65) to the number under this age. According to data from the United Nations, the OADR in the UK is currently about 310 (that is, 310 people over state pension age to every 1000 people age 20-64). Although it has been fairly constant since the 1980s, it has begun to rise steadily since 2010 as the early boomers reach state pension age. Current projections suggest it could rise to 480 by 2050.[41] It is suggested that the 'ideal dependency ratio' is about four workers for every retiree, which is an OADR of 250, so we are already breaching this 'ideal' number. This is seen as a major problem for public sector finances.

The traditional calculation of OADR is a really blunt measure. It essentially counts everyone over 65 as economically 'dependent', i.e. not working or contributing productively to the economy, and assumes that everyone below 65 is working, paying taxes and contributing to the economy. Because of this, it's not a good measure to understand what's going on.

SINGAPORE'S PLAN FOR SUCCESSFUL AGEING

Singapore's *Action Plan for Successful Ageing* was developed in 2015, after extensive consultation with its older population, and resulted in 70 initiatives in 12 areas to make Singapore more age-friendly. Areas such as employment, educational opportunities and health care were all raised as important issues for the older population.

Amongst the key initiatives and targets were government commitments to helping people work for longer if they want, and are able, to do so. To support this, the government also pledged to create a new workplace health programme for more than 120,000 people over 40 to help them stay healthy. Other initiatives included: a National Silver Academy to allow older people to pursue further learning; the expansion of home nursing care; improving the accessibility of the built environment; and the recruitment of 50,000 older volunteers. The government estimated that the cost of these programmes to prepare Singapore for 'successful ageing' was in the region of $3 billion (SGD).

Although many of these initiatives were aimed at improving daily life for older people in Singapore, the Maintenance of Parents Act also provides legal recourse for older parents who are not being financially supported by their children.[42]

Not everyone of working age is working: in July 2019, 29% of 18 to 24-year-olds were economically inactive. And not everyone beyond state pension age is economically inactive: in fact, 11% of over 65s were in work. That means that 1.3 million people were working beyond the age of 65.[43] If the point is to understand the pressures on public finances that arise when fewer people are paying taxes (contributors) and more people are relying on public spending (beneficiaries), then why not have a dependency ratio for the whole population, regardless of age, comparing the number of contributors to the number of beneficiaries?

This would still fail to account for the economic contribution of those who are not in paid work. The indirect economic contribution of those caring for others is not insignificant. The gross value added of unpaid care for adult relatives or spouses has been estimated at £59.5 billion and grandparents are providing childcare worth £6.6 billion,[44] often enabling women who would otherwise not have returned to work to participate in paid work.[45]

Given gains in life expectancy at older ages, changes in health status at different ages and changes in the economic activity of those over 65, OADR is no longer a useful way of looking at the changing population age profile. Rather than use chronological age (time from birth), a better way to look at this is to calculate how many years one can expect to have left to live (time from death). This prospective old age dependency ratio (POADR) usually measures how many people there are with a remaining life expectancy of 15 years or less, compared to those over 20 years of age who are expected to live longer than 15 years. Using this measure, the UK's POADR is projected to rise from 173 for every 1000 people in 2015 to 227 per 1000 people in 2050. This is much lower than the conventional OADR measure, which is projected to increase from 310 to 480 per 1000 people in the same time period.[46] So overall this is a much less worrying picture than that painted by the conventional way of measuring this.

As we will see in the next chapter, OADR is commonly used by those wanting to paint a doomsday scenario that there are too many older people to be supported by the younger working population. It is usually wheeled out to justify reforms to public pensions or to suggest that publicly funded health and long-term care are 'unsustainable'. While clearly there are going to be some challenges associated with such a dramatic age shift in the population, these need not be insurmountable.

In this chapter we have seen the dramatic age shift that is occurring in our society. Our longer lives are one of the greatest achievements of public health and medical science. The consequence of such a rapid increase in life span at the same time as the largest surviving birth cohort in the last hundred years is turning 60 is that the face of our society is changing. Old age is becoming the new normal. This is one of the most profound changes in human history and yet it seems to have crept up on us. This is not a problem that is way off in the future. It is right here, right now. It is us. It is our parents. It is our grandparents. The rising numbers of older people are an inevitability, but the consequences for society are not. As we will see in the next chapter, some predict dire consequences. Are they right to and what, if anything, can we do to change the course of history?

2

We're all doomed

'Our fears about our society and the strains in our economy reflect a breakdown in the balance between the generations. It is under threat from the [post-war] baby boomers ... not because of deliberate selfishness but because of their sheer demographic and economic power. Younger generations are losing out.'[1]

David Willetts, *The Pinch*

The fact that we are living longer should be good news and yet the prevailing narrative is one which depicts later life as a time of decline and misery (see box on page 26). The cult of youth prevails, with adverts promoting beauty products that are 'anti-ageing' and recruiters seeking 'fresh talent'. The age shift in the population is seen as an impending disaster. The fear is that we are going to be overwhelmed by a 'tsunami' of older people; that rising pension and health care costs are going to break the bank. Everything from levels of national debt to the fact that young people are being squeezed out of the housing market is blamed on the growing numbers of older people. The debate about falling living standards is used to fuel intergenerational conflict, pitting old against young. Are we heading for a dystopian future, a society in which the fault lines are no longer based on gender, race or class, but instead on age?

RECENT HEADLINES ABOUT OUR AGEING POPULATION

'Britain's age timebomb: Cost of 1.4 million extra pensioners "means NHS cannot stay free"'[2]

'Britain faces old age poverty timebomb as one in five put NOTHING in a pension'[3]

'Britain needs millions more immigrants to reduce strain of ageing population'[4]

'National debt will hit unsustainable levels by 2060s because of rising elderly population says watchdog'.[5]

THE WORST TIME OF YOUR LIFE: ATTITUDES TO AGE AND AGEISM

We are bombarded daily with conflicting and inflammatory reports about what it is to grow older in today's world. Recent stories in the British media have included: whether restrictions should be imposed on older drivers after Prince Phillip's high-profile car accident; sensational coverage of Joyce Williams, the octogenarian blogger who has written about sex in later life; and puzzlement at the story of 88-year-old Eileen Jolly, the NHS worker who successfully sued the NHS for age discrimination. However, for a multitude of reasons we are yet to see fair and meaningful depictions of ageing in the media, advertising or cultural spheres. Stereotyping and casual ageism remain rife.

Adverts featuring older consumers create and reinforce stereotypes. A TV advert for a property website depicts an older man seen going up and down stairs carrying various items, including a tool box, a box of Christmas decorations and a breakfast tray. He then disappears from his family home of many years to make way for a younger family. The final shot is of him putting up photos in his new bungalow, reinforcing the idea that old people should downsize and live in a bungalow. (As we will see in the chapter on housing, this is both unrealistic and not what older people themselves want). Older adults are invisible or incidental in general adverts. Where they do feature it is often in ads for specialist products (incontinence pads, stair lifts, home adaptations, etc.). Images of older people in ads are somewhat idealistic, presenting the 'golden ager' as generally more affluent or the 'perfect grandparent'.[6]

Later life is framed as something to be endured rather than enjoyed. Ageism is pernicious and the responsibility falls to every one of us to recognise it and to call it out. Everyday ageism is on display when you go to buy a birthday card. Jokes about being over the hill are still the staple, although if you're lucky you might find one that equates getting old with a good wine or cheese that gets better with age. We also internalise these attitudes and place limits on ourselves, saying, 'I really shouldn't at my age.' When we forget someone's name we say we are 'having a senior moment'. We blame our age for those nagging aches and pains. These insidious words and phrases equate getting older with don'ts, decline, dementia and disease. It is little wonder then that we fear it. Language reinforces and shapes our attitudes.

Unfortunately, such attitudes are pervasive. In a 2018 survey of 2000 people of all ages conducted by the Royal Society for Public Health and the Calouste Gulbenkian Foundation, a quarter of 18 to 34-year-olds thought that older people can never be considered attractive and a quarter thought it was normal to be unhappy and depressed when you are in old age. It is testament to those campaigning for greater awareness of dementia that this is now widely understood by young and old. However, perceptions are such that young people today assume that all old people have dementia. Two-fifths of young people in the above survey thought that there's no way to avoid getting dementia in later life.[7]

A number of global surveys by Ipsos Mori have demonstrated there are significant misconceptions about the age shift. In 2014, the average British respondent under 65 thought that 37% of the population was over 65, when it was in fact only

17%.[8] Furthermore, when it came to expectations of later life, the British were among the least optimistic when people in 29 countries were questioned in another Ipsos Mori survey. Only 38% of British respondents, who were all under 65, agreed with the statement, 'I expect to be fit and healthy when I grow old,' compared to a global average of 57% and an overwhelming majority of Colombian respondents (89%).[9]

Think for a minute about all the terms we have to describe the 30% of the population who are under the age of 25: baby, infant, toddler, pre-schooler, child, pupil, teenager, young person, student. While there are a range of terms used to describe those over the age of 65, these range from administrative terms, such as old age pensioner and senior citizen, to insulting or at best patronising terms, such as old codger, old fogey, golden oldie and old timer, to terms that marketers have invented, such as silver surfers. We demean the older age group in our language and yet when it comes to debates about fairness the older generation are caricatured as 'having it all'. The image is of someone spending their retirement sailing around the world on a cruise ship or playing golf, spending the kids' inheritance, enjoying a generous final salary pension and, having made a killing on the housing market when times were good, living in a large house with more rooms than they could possibly find a use for.

So what is a more realistic way to understand the differences among older generations? The Centre for Ageing Better commissioned research which analysed data from the English Longitudinal Study of Ageing to segment the population over 50 years old into six groups based on wellbeing scores and other factors.[10] Unlike most analyses, they are not neatly based on age, although the two groups called boomers were more likely to be in their 60s at the time the data were collected in 2012, which means they were born between 1943 and 1952, around the post-World War II baby boom.

INTRODUCING THE LATER LIFE STUDY POPULATION SEGMENTS

Thriving boomers: While not true of everyone in this segment, they are more likely to be in their 60s and living with a partner. While they may have children, they are likely to have left home, giving these people time and space. They're likely to be retired and, as they have paid off their mortgage, they have more disposable income that they can spend on holidays, and social and cultural activities. They have a strong network of family, friends and people they feel they can rely on – all of which contribute to high levels of wellbeing. They make up 21% of people in the sample and have higher than average reported levels of happiness. I'll introduce you to Simon aged 69 and retired, one of the people interviewed as part of the study, who is typical of this group. He is fit and healthy, enjoys holidays and time with his family.

Downbeat boomers: This segment is similar demographically to the thriving boomers, but very different in their outlook. While not the case for all in this segment, these people are likely to be in their 60s and in a stable relationship. They are well-educated and have had a good career – something which has contributed to their positive financial situation. They're in good health and participate socially, but in spite of all this they are not as satisfied with their life as others in similar circumstances. They again make up 21% of people in the sample, but only one in 10 of this group reported feeling very happy the day before the survey. Qualitative interviews suggested that this group are more likely to reflect on missed opportunities or what they could have done differently. I'll highlight the experiences of Kate, who is typical of this group. She is 63, healthy and active. However, the loss of her parents has hit her hard, and she is worried about her own future and later life.

Can do and connected: While this description does not match all those in this segment, they are more likely to be women aged

70 and over who are single or widowed. Now retired, they spent their working lives in low skilled work, looking after the home or raising children. They don't have a lot of money and sometimes struggle to pay for all the things they need. Their health is also starting to limit what they can do, but to them this is just a part of getting older. They feel lucky to have people they can call on for help and support and are content with their lives. They recognise that things could be a lot worse. This group makes up 19% of the sample. Mary, whose story I'll share, is fairly typical of this group. She is 76 and a widow. Despite a number of health problems, she is extremely active in her local community and sees friends regularly.

Worried and disconnected: While not true of all those in this segment, who constitute 13% of the sample, these people are typically similar demographically to those classed as 'can do and connected', but with weaker social connections and a more negative outlook on later life. They are older, aged 70 or above, and have retired. The house where they live is increasingly unsuitable for them and they may have made some changes to it to address this. They feel isolated – they need people more than they used to, but don't want to be a burden. They have enough money to spend on their needs, including the odd treat, but find that going out is more difficult, which adds to their sense of loneliness. James, who is typical of this group, is 71 and a retired long-distance lorry driver. He has several chronic conditions and, since he lost his partner, he spends time alone at home.

Squeezed middle-age: While not true of all in this segment, these people, who make up 14% of our sample, are predominantly in their 50s and typically married or living with a partner. They are more likely to be in good health than average. They also are mostly working full-time – retirement seems like a long way off. They may have children still living at home and, on top of this, may have to provide care for their own parents. This puts them under both time and financial pressures, leaving them feeling less in control compared to others and less able to maintain social relationships. This pressure on resources also means they are more likely than average to lack the money they need to meet their needs and a third (33%) report low happiness scores. This is the group who are most likely to be born during the 1960s baby boom. Rachel is 52 and has a job, but juggles this with caring for her mother with dementia. She has two children living at home, with one away at university. She faces some of the challenges typical of this group.

Struggling and alone: This segment, who are 12% of our sample, are distributed across the age range, but are most likely to be aged 50-59 or 80+. While not the case for all in this segment, many of them live on their own. While some own their own home, some still rent, which is a significant drain on their finances, and they often find they're short of money at the end of each month. They are less likely than average to have enough money for their needs and are more likely to be in poverty. Many have a long-standing illness and suffer with frequent pain, which affects every aspect of their life. They're also socially isolated, which makes them feel dissatisfied with their life. Trevor, who we'll meet later, is 59, has serious back problems, is no longer working and also has depression.

Throughout this book I'll be using case studies of people from these six groups to illustrate experiences common to people within these groups. These segments highlight the breadth and diversity that exists among people over 50 in the UK. In fact, only a small minority (about 21%) of those over 50 are in the group of thriving boomers and fit the classic stereotype of someone financially secure, in good health and enjoying life to the full. As we will see, there are deep seated inequalities among people in later life due to socio-economic status, ethnicity, gender and where people live.

Older people are not necessarily overtly demonised and are often perceived as kind or warm. However, they are also stereotyped as being a financial and social burden, incompetent and unproductive.[11] In a survey of 16 to 64-year-olds, more than a third of respondents considered people in old age to be

31

wise. A similar proportion also thought older people were frail and lonely. This has been described as the 'doddery but dear' archetype, i.e. lacking in competence but friendly.[12]

You could ask what is the problem with these attitudes? Surely every generation has stereotypes about other generations. Isn't there just as much ageism towards young people as there is towards older people? While stereotypes have their uses – they help us to understand the world, providing us with rules of thumb which help to simplify what would otherwise be an overload of information – they can also be used to discriminate. Age discrimination is illegal under the Equality Act 2010. There is some evidence to suggest that older patients do not get the same access to health care as younger patients and that older workers face age discrimination in the workplace. Despite this, very few cases have been brought on the basis of age.

Zoe Wyrko, a doctor who specialises in the care of older people and who appeared on the TV show *Old People's Home for 4 Year Olds,* is critical of our conflicting attitudes to old age: 'If someone is in their 90s, someone else might say, "Oh isn't that great. Isn't that fabulous. Let's celebrate that long life." But then that same person will be ageist and discriminatory in another context. We need to reconsider that; it can't be both things.' Negative attitudes among health professionals can affect decisions to treat, with older patients receiving lower treatment rates and reduced access to surgery on the basis of their age.[13] Wyrko suggests that doctors are getting around anti-discrimination rules by using frailty instead of age: 'They know they can't discriminate because of people's age or shouldn't, so instead they're just saying they're frail, with no grounds for that whatsoever. It's the new ageism.'

Age discrimination is also common in the workplace. A Centre for Ageing Better survey of 1,100 employees aged over 50 found that over one in 10 said they have had comments or jokes made about their age in their current job. As well as this, one in five thinks that people view them as less capable at work as they get older.[14]

Depending on how old you currently are, this form of discrimination and prejudice is not only something you may be experiencing now, but something that we may all experience in the future. Widely held cultural stereotypes of older people can become internalised over the life course. For example, the negative stereotype that portrays older people as less able physically and cognitively actually results in older people being less willing to engage in physical activity and is associated with poorer physical health and lower cognitive functioning.[15] It can lead people to self-censor and not put themselves forward for certain jobs or leadership opportunities. If they perceive they don't fit, or the organisation and co-workers do not respect or appreciate older workers, they are more likely to intend to leave work.[16]

Ageism, just like other isms, makes people feel bad about themselves and has detrimental effects on our health and wellbeing. We know that people internalise experiences of ageism and these in turn impact how old they feel.[17] It is not only perception; physical functioning is also demonstrably better among those who feel younger, so our outlook really matters to our health.[18]

The former Director of Ageing and Life Course at the World Health Organisation, Dr John Beard, sees ageism as a huge problem in health care: 'The fundamental problem is ageism, and stereotyping people on the basis of chronological age. These stereotypes are usually based on how people's health was at that age many years ago and perpetually frames problems as though we're living in the past. Consequently, the solutions are relevant to the past, not the future.'

Such negative associations with later life not only reinforce stereotypes and prejudice between generations, but they also make us fear our future selves. This leads to denial and can result in people acting fatalistically and not taking action to prepare or plan for later life. Those without high-value assets, often private renters or those in low-earning jobs, are even less likely to make plans for their future and do not feel it is within their power to do so.[19]

It is perhaps then little surprise that most of us are in denial, given that negative attitudes towards old age are pervasive in our society. We are often encouraged to look to countries like Japan, which have more older people and who are living longer on average than other countries, to understand how we should respond. And yet only 1 in 10 Japanese people are looking forward to their own old age and nearly 9 in 10 see the ageing population as a major problem.[20]

The negative language we use cultivates negative attitudes and reinforces stereotypes. These not only impact on us as individuals, but also distort how decision-makers respond to the age shift. The extent of age stereotypes and the failure to acknowledge that chronological age is a very poor indicator of a person's needs can result in a failed public policy response. Let's look next at the how the economists portray the impact of the dramatic shift in the age profile of the population. Are we set to face economic catastrophe as a direct result of the big age shift?

ECONOMIC DISASTER: IS THE AGE SHIFT A THREAT TO THE ECONOMY?

Most ministries of finance, like the Treasury here in the UK, worry about the fiscal challenge of an ageing population. Much of the focus of governments in developed welfare states is on the sustainability or otherwise of the pension systems, and the affordability of health and long-term care systems. In the UK, where social care is funded locally, these worries are often shared by local leaders who see the pressure on social care budgets that result from more people living longer. Looked at this way, the ageing population is seen as a fiscal risk to sustainability.

The Office for Budgetary Responsibility (OBR) provides independent analysis of the UK's public finances, including forecasting the performance of the economy, as well as public spending. In July 2017 it published its first analysis of fiscal risks, setting out the issues which are likely to pose the greatest threats to the future of the public finances in the UK. Among the highest risks? Population ageing.

The OBR sets out the risk as follows: 'The ageing of the population is the most important demographic factor over the medium- and longer-term – specifically the number of elderly adults

34

as a percentage of those of working-age (the "old age dependency ratio"). This is the key driver of spending as a share of GDP and the most important demand-side driver of pensions spending (as well as on health and social care).' There's that measure again – the OADR – that we critiqued in the first chapter. While the OBR goes on to suggest that many of the risks set out would have been apparent in an assessment made at any time over the past 30 years – suggesting many of the drivers of public spending remain the same for some head-in-the-sand reason – the 'pressures of ageing', as it calls them, have 'risen in prominence more recently'. While health spending driven by other cost pressures (such as technology) is rated by the OBR as having a higher impact on public finances than increases in health and adult social care spending driven by ageing, the probability of these age-related risks actually occurring is very likely (over 90% chance of the risk crystallising). Given that these people are already alive, it is almost certain that this issue will need to be faced.[21]

From the perspective of the Treasury the projected increases in public expenditure on pensions, and health and social care, pose a threat to its ability to balance the books. If the current limits being placed on levels of borrowing and debt continue, any increases in expenditure will have to be met by reductions in other areas of spending (already stripped back through repeated rounds of cuts, for example to education) or increasing revenues (through tax rises or increases to National Insurance contributions). Treasury officials look at graphs, like the one on page 36, which shows the profile of tax contributions and public expenditure by age and conclude that the growing numbers of people at older ages relative to those of working age is a disaster.

The graph shows that children and older people are net beneficiaries while those of working age are net contributors. This means that at any point in time there are transfers between generations from those aged between 20 and 65 years old to those over 65. However, it is also possible to look at the contributions we each make over our lifetime and view the distribution below as smoothing out across the life course. These arguments are central to the debate about the so-called intergenerational contract – the principle that different generations support each other across the different stages of their lives. I explore this further below.

From the point of view of the state this balance comes under greater strain when the numbers of net contributors relative to the number of net beneficiaries falls, as represented by the old age dependency ratio, which currently suggests there are three over 65s for every 10 working age adults. David Willetts, former Conservative MP, argued in his influential book *The Pinch* that the state can play a positive role in maintaining a 'fair' balance, but there is a risk it is hijacked by a particular generation's interests: 'At its best government helps maintain the balance between the generations and helps shift resources between the different stages of the life cycle in a way that complements what families do. However, it can instead allow itself to be captured by particular generational interests that exploit this power.'[22] An example of this might be older generations preserving more generous pension entitlements while eroding working age benefits.

None of the options to rebalance this look very palatable (at least not politically); for example, pushing the 'tax' curve to the

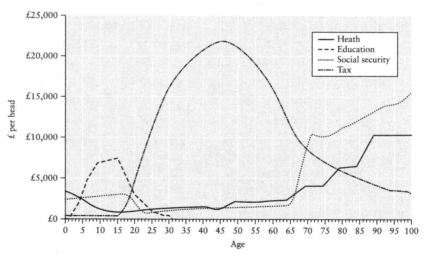

Projected average spend and tax revenue per head and area of provision by age 2021-22.

Source: Resolution Foundation (2019) RF analysis of Office of Budget Responsibility's Fiscal Sustainability Report.

right by increasing National Insurance and tax contributions at older ages, or increasing Inheritance Tax or other wealth taxes. Currently some older adults who are working are exempt from contributing to certain taxes, e.g. National Insurance. Some of those with large amounts of wealth avoid paying Inheritance Tax. Tax treatment of pension income means that pensioners pay less than those of working age on similar incomes. For those in work after they qualify for their pension, their National Insurance exemption and tax-free state pension (assuming full entitlement) could give an income boost of more than £226 a week compared to someone under pension age earning the same amount.[23]

Other proposals to shift this balance are met with opposition, too. The main objection to increases in Inheritance Tax seems to be a view that this wealth is a right of future generations. There is a strongly held view that it is one's right to pass on one's home (or at least the housing wealth) to one's children (or grandchildren). But this locks these wealth assets within families, limiting redistribution and reinforcing inequalities across generations. As inheritances get bigger due to the accumulation of wealth in property, the risk is that the inequalities in the older generations will perpetuate inequalities in subsequent generations.

Some action is being taken to push the 'social security' line to the right by delaying the age at which pensions are paid. However, other options, such as reducing the value of those pensions or changing who is eligible are less acceptable, as we will see in the next chapter, on money. Rapid increases in the state pension age for women to equalise it with the state pension age for men have left a group of women born in the 1950s unprepared for a longer period until they can draw their state pension. About 300,000 women born between 6 December 1953 and 5 October 1954 have, or are expected to, wait 18 months longer to collect their pensions.[24] They are angry and large numbers have mobilised as Women Against State Pension Age Increases (WASPI). They have taken their case to the courts, claiming that the government ignored recommendations that it phase in the changes much more slowly, and also that women directly affected were given little or no notice about the impending changes. Any government that makes radical changes to the 'sacred cow' of the state pension has to be prepared to face the wrath of angry pensioners.

And universal age-related benefits such as free TV licenses, bus passes and winter fuel payments are a visible target, with opponents pointing out that they are given to wealthy pensioners while those struggling on low incomes at younger ages have to pay for these costs. Proposals to remove such benefits from pensioners, while they grab the headlines, have little impact on the overall costs. For example, when the BBC recently announced their decision to end free TV licenses for all but the poorest over-75s, this generated a backlash from pensioner groups. A recent House of Lords Select Committee on intergenerational fairness recommended a number of changes, including means testing a number of universal pensioner benefits, such as Winter Fuel Payment. It also called for government to abolish the triple lock – the mechanism for increasing the value of the state pension each year – in favour of uprating the state pension in line with increases in average wages. The committee was clear that the tax and benefit system as it stands is not awake to the reality of our longer lives.[25]

Other strategies to contain spending by reducing expenditure on health and social care (the solid black line), for example, by reducing demand through actions to prevent ill health or reducing the 'offer' of what treatments are provided and to whom, are seen to be uncertain or unacceptable respectively. I'll look at some of the options for reducing health and social care spending in chapters 6 and 7.

Clearly the age shift does impact on public spending, but the simple interpretation that this is an unsustainable burden and will inevitably lead to problems for society is wrong. As you will discover in this book, we do have choices. These are not easy choices, but if we face up to reality and start to take action now, we can change our future for the better. The challenge is how to get public and political support for these changes when so much of the debate is framed in terms of old versus young.

IS INTERGENERATIONAL CONFLICT ON THE RISE?

The plight of the millennials is blamed on older generations. The baby boomers' fortune is at the expense of future generations: drawing their generous pensions and bankrupting pension funds so there's nothing left; living in their big houses worth hundreds of thousands of pounds, putting the prospects of home ownership way beyond the reach of a first-time buyer; and enjoying life's luxuries while young people are having to cut back on non-essentials such as eating out. These intergenerational divisions also extend to wider issues, such as the environment and politics. The climate emergency is blamed on older generations: they are responsible for plundering the world's resources, carbon emissions from fossil fuels and for leaving the planet polluted for generations to come. The older generations have also been 'blamed' for voting to leave the European Union, denying young people opportunities to study and work in other European countries, and leaving them to deal with the long-term economic consequences. Although analysis of polling data suggests that approximately 55% of those over 55 voted to leave, there is a stronger link between voting leave and education, geography, socio-economic factors and feeling 'English' than with age.[26]

Perhaps these beliefs many voice – whether correct or not – are not surprising, because we know few people of other ages. Society is age-segregated. Most of our relationships are horizontal, that is with people of a similar age to ourselves. Very few of the respondents to a recent survey had intergenerational friendships and barely a third had friendships with those three or more decades older than themselves.[27]

David Willetts, in *The Pinch*, posited that the intergenerational contract is under threat. He argues that the accumulation of economic, social and political power by the [post-war] baby boomers puts at risk the prosperity of future generations. He argues that being 'a big generation gives you a lot of power. Your large cohort will dominate marketplaces. You will be kings and queens amongst consumers. Elections will be pitched to you. In fact, your

.

values and tastes will shape the world around you – you will be able to spend your life in a generational bubble, always outvoting and outspending the generations before and after you. That is what it means to be a baby boomer.'[28] He cites evidence that the next generation's living standards will not match those of previous generations, as home ownership levels fall, house prices rise, debt levels increase, pension benefits reduce and the prospect of a secure job for life disappears with changes in the nature of work.

Willetts is now Chair of the Resolution Foundation, a think-tank focused on living standards for those on low to middle incomes. It is largely funded by the Resolution Trust, which was started with £50 million from the founder of the investment and insurance firm of the same name. Willetts chaired their Intergenerational Commission, set up in 2016 to look at the drivers of different living standards within and between generations. The Commission documents how the experiences of various life stages differ between generations to understand whether, and how, living standards are changing over time. While employment rates are high, pay has stagnated, due to poor wage growth following the financial crisis, and work tends to be less secure than it was. Home ownership rates are much lower than for previous generations at the same age, and the lack of social housing means a huge rise in the proportion in private rented accommodation – which is often smaller, less secure and in poorer condition – and housing consumes a higher proportion of income. Although each generation has generally earned more than the last at age 25, the gains seem to be smaller with each successive cohort and came to a halt in the early 2000s. Millennials (born 1981-2000) are less likely to own their own homes and less likely to move jobs, slowing wage progression.[29]

It appears things are changing and successive generations are being impacted more heavily by austerity, the squeeze on living standards, triple-digit house price rises and the changing nature of the labour market. However, joint analysis by the Centre for Ageing Better and Resolution Foundation found that this is not just limited to younger generations. About 1.8 million people between 50 and state pension age live in low-to-middle income households, nearly a third of all such households. These are in the bottom half of the income distribution but with income above the bottom 10% and less than a fifth of their income from means-tested benefits. The living standards of older people on low-to-middle incomes are no higher than they were in 2007-2008.[30] So it is perhaps no surprise that, as a nation, we have become decidedly pessimistic about the future; those who believe that young adults' chances of having higher living standards than their parents are outnumbered by two to one by the pessimists. This is a rapid reversal from 2003, when optimists outnumbered pessimists by nearly four to one.[31] What is this future that these pessimists envisage? Let's try and imagine the dystopia created by the age shift if we do nothing.

THE AGE OF AGEING BADLY

Let me take you to the world of ageing badly, a dystopian future circa 2040, only 20 years from now. Technological advances have accelerated, resulting in the widespread automation of jobs. There are high unemployment rates and fewer people contributing taxes. Employment rights have been steadily eroded as more people shift onto part-time and flexible contracts. As a result, those with disabilities and health conditions are finding it harder to remain in work, with employers unwilling to make adjustments. Fewer workers are contributing to pensions, more have opted out as contribution rates have increased and the numbers of self-employed have risen. The FAANGs – Facebook, Amazon, Apple, Netflix and Google – have got their teeth into every aspect of our lives, dominating markets and eluding the national tax authorities. Tax revenues have plummeted and as a result there have been further public spending cuts.

The state pension has been further reduced and for the first time in 50 years the NHS has had a real-terms cut in its budget for five years running. A further wave of local authorities has declared themselves bankrupt, unable to meet their statutory responsibilities, having run out of money. The social care reforms introduced in 2021 were never properly implemented and families are having to provide care for their relatives. Those with private pension savings are struggling financially, because of poor economic performance and very low returns.

Corporatisation and the convenience of virtual shops and drone deliveries means the high streets and shopping malls are empty. Communities have become unsafe and green spaces are no-go areas for people of all ages. Public transport has all but disappeared as fewer people travel to towns to shop or commute to work as jobs have disappeared or changed, with more people working remotely at computers or in large out-of-town warehouses. People of different ages rarely mix. Fear and suspicion are rife between generations, fuelled by negative social media campaigns and divisive political rhetoric.

Obesity rates and high levels of depression have resulted in a reversal in life expectancy gains and there are high levels of disability among older adults. Poor quality and poorly designed housing built during the housing boom in the early 2020s means more older people are housebound and there were record deaths from heat exhaustion during the previous summer's extreme temperatures. Housing built in the last century is in disrepair, as older low-income owner-occupiers can't afford to keep up with maintenance and rising energy and heating bills. There are more private renters living in poor quality housing and landlords refuse to adapt properties to enable older people to live independently. Consequently, there are higher rates of hospital and care admissions.

Is this what's waiting for us in 20 years? It doesn't have to be this way. While there are challenges, not least the ageist views and attitudes described here, and the pressures on public finances from pensions, and health and social care spending, my aim is to unpack the facts, bust a few myths and set out a different path, one that leads to a more positive future – the world of ageing better. Let's kick off by looking at one of the most financially challenging issues we face as a consequence of the age shift – pensions.

3

Money, money, money

"A workman who has contributed health and strength, vigour
and skill, to the creation of wealth by which taxation is borne
has made his contribution already to the fund which is to give
him a pension when he is no longer fit to create that wealth."[1]

David Lloyd George, Hansard, June 1908

Pensions have been the main method of providing an income
in old age since their introduction in Europe in the late 1800s.
Before the introduction of pensions, old age was associated with
destitution and poverty. Many of those who were unable to work,
and whose families could not support them, were admitted to the
workhouses.[2] By the late 1880s the vast majority of people in the
poorhouses and workhouses were older people.

Many of the early pension schemes were voluntary contributory
schemes run by charities and friendly societies. Friendly societies
were for many years strongly opposed to the introduction of a
national contributory pension as many higher paid workers were
members of friendly societies, which entitled them to sick pay
and a funeral allowance. A state insurance system threatened
their financial viability. Nevertheless, the first state pension was
introduced in the UK by Prime Minister Herbert Asquith's Liberal
government in 1908. It was a means-tested benefit for men over
70 who had been resident for at least 20 years and passed certain
behavioural tests. At the time a man's average life expectancy was
only 55, so the majority of people were dead before they ever

received the pension.[3] Today, on average people spend a third of their life in retirement and current policy is that state pension age should increase to keep this proportion constant. You can see the challenge. Can we afford to support the growing numbers of people in old age to spend a third of their lives in retirement? Is the age shift going to bankrupt us and leave more of us living our later life in poverty?

In this chapter I'll explore the role of the state in ensuring we have financial security in old age and how this has changed over time. I'll look at the affordability of the state pension: who should get it and how much should they get? At what age should people receive it? And should it remain universal or do we need to consider means-testing?

Relying on the state pension is unlikely to be sufficient for most people – the new state pension, introduced in April 2016, was at time of writing £168.60 a week for those who receive the full amount. Private and occupational pensions, therefore, play an increasingly important role in ensuring a reasonable standard of living in old age. And yet traditional occupational pension funds are effectively 'bankrupt', with obligations to pay pensions for existing members outstripping the amount held in the fund and employers unable to make extra payments to cover this. Many schemes have closed to new members or changed radically, so they put a lot more responsibility on the individual and no longer guarantee an amount that they will pay out. Making our own saving plans, then, is essential.

But planning our future finances is difficult and the array of choices bewildering. I once heard someone suggest that in order to make these decisions we need to be an actuary (to predict how long we will live), a careers adviser (to understand how we can keep working for longer), a financial adviser (to assess our financial requirements), an investment broker (to decide where to invest our money to get the best returns) and a clairvoyant (to see into the future and what will happen in our lives). A pretty tall order for anyone!

For all the talk of rich pensioners enjoying retirement on a generous pension, there are estimated to be 2 million pensioners living in relative poverty, meaning their income is less than 60% of the median income (in that year) after housing costs. 1.6 million of these are pensioners are also in absolute poverty, meaning their income is less than 60% of what the median income was in a fixed year (2010/11 is often used) after accounting for housing costs. This measure allows us to use a 'fixed' standard of low income, rather than just measuring against how everyone else is doing. While pensioner poverty has been falling over the last decade, there are worrying signs that progress on pensioner poverty is reversing: 2017-2018 saw the first rise in more than a decade.[4]

The fact is that many of us are not saving enough (or anything at all). If we are to ensure that everyone has enough to live off in old age, we have to radically rethink personal savings and the role of the state in ensuring we are better prepared. There is a real risk that if we don't do something urgently, the reductions in pensioner poverty that we have seen over the last decade will go into reverse.

CAN WE AFFORD THE STATE PENSION?

The main argument put forward by the doom-mongers is that in future years the state pension will bankrupt the Treasury. The question is framed as one of affordability: more older people means higher expenditure on the state pension; relatively fewer people of working age means not enough tax revenues to pay for it. When there is a big birth cohort in retirement, as is happening now with the first wave of baby boomers, then tax-payers right now have to pay more to fund the increase in the pension bill. This is seen as creating an 'unfair' burden on working age adults. The other age-related benefits, such as Winter Fuel Payment, free TV licenses and free bus passes, also get brought into the debate about intergenerational fairness. While these benefits do have a financial cost to the state, as well as a value to the beneficiaries, they are dwarfed by the cost of the state pension itself, so here I'll stick with a focus on pensions.

Projections by the Office of Budget Responsibility (OBR) suggest that state pensions will increase from 5.1% of GDP currently to 6.9% of GDP over the next 50 years (given current policies). This is modest compared to the predicted growth in health care costs, which are set to nearly double from 7.1% of GDP in 2017-2018 to 13.8% over the next 50 years.[5] I'll come back to the concerns about health care spending in the next chapter and look at how much this is caused by the age shift.

The state pension, looked at in this way, as a question of affordability for working age taxpayers, leads policy makers to ask questions such as is the state pension too generous? Should the rate at which the value of the state pension is increased each year be reduced? Should the age at which people receive the state pension increase? And, more radically, should the pension no longer be universal, thereby reducing the number of people eligible for the state pension? In other words, can the state pay less to fewer people and for less time? Let's look at each of these issues in turn before we continue our search for better solutions.

HOW MUCH SHOULD THE STATE PENSION BE?

The way that the debate is framed suggests the state pension is providing everyone with a decent amount to live off. This is far from the truth. Let's have a look at how much people are actually getting.

For those retiring since April 2016, the new state pension provides a flat-rate amount (i.e. it isn't earnings related). The actual amount an individual receives depends on the number of years they have made (or been credited with) National Insurance contributions. To get the full amount, which in 2019-2020 was £168.60 a week, you need 35 qualifying years and at least 10 years to get anything at all. Those not receiving the full state pension (due to having fewer qualifying years) could be eligible to receive means-tested Pension Credit, a top-up benefit which guarantees a minimum income, currently £167.25 for a single person. However, of those eligible for Pension Credit only 60% actually claim.[6] This is because the means-tested system, based on income and earnings, is both complex and stigmatising and so people forego the financial support to which they are entitled.

Those retiring before April 2016 were eligible for a basic state pension which required 30 qualifying years to receive a full state pension. In addition, up until 2002, they might have contributed to an additional state pension, known as the State Earnings Related Pension Scheme (SERPS), which was replaced by the State Second Pension between 2002 and 2016. From 1978 to 2016 it was possible to pay additional contributions to receive an earnings-related state pension. This created an incentive to contribute more in order to receive a higher state pension. The UK is one of very few countries in which there is no longer a link between an individual's previous earnings and the amount they get in state pension income. Since the introduction of the new flat rate state pension in 2016 the percentage of previous earnings that most people will receive in retirement, if they rely on the UK state pension alone, will not exceed 30%. This compares to an average of 63% in the Organisation for Economic Co-operation and Development (OECD) nations, where the link between earnings and state pension entitlements continues in many countries.[7] As we will see, in the UK it means greater reliance on private and occupational pensions to provide more than a basic income in old age. It also suggests that any further erosion of the value of the state pension would put us in a league with much less prosperous countries.

The value of the state pension has been much debated. After the link with earnings was broken in the 1980s and the state pension was tied instead to inflation, its value fell relative to average earnings. In 1979, for example, the basic state pension was 26% of national average earnings. This fell to just 16.3% in 2010.[8] Rates of pensioner poverty reduced significantly between the mid-1990s and early 2010s, largely due to increases in income from private and occupational pensions, and benefits such as Pension Credit, rather than any increases in the state pension.[9] From 2011, the annual increases in the value of the state pension were 'triple-locked' – they were tied to inflation, average earnings or 2.5%, whichever was the greatest. This has restored the basic state pension to over 18% of national average earnings, while the more generous new state pension is 24% of national average earnings in 2019.[10] Critics have argued that the government should abandon the triple lock and reduce the value of the pension, but that risks increasing poverty.

The triple lock was specifically introduced in 2011 as part of a package of measures by the Coalition Government to increase the value of the pension to ensure it was 'decent' and 'properly indexed' at a time when the state pension age was increasing. There are calls now to remove the triple lock and to replace it with either an earnings inflation link or a 'double lock', which would increase the state pension by whichever is higher – earnings or inflation. Analysis by the Pensions Policy Institute (PPI), an independent policy and research organisation, suggested that the number of pensioners in poverty would increase by 1% by 2050 if the triple lock was replaced with a double lock, and 4% if it were replaced with an earnings inflation link, equivalent to an additional 200,000 or 700,000 pensioners in poverty respectively.[11]

Recent data has shown that these guaranteed rises in the value of the state pension have resulted in the median income of retired households, after taxes, rising faster than that of working and non-retired households.[12] At the same time a four-year freeze on most working age benefits and tax credits introduced in 2015 has meant income has fallen behind the rising cost of living. According to the Joseph Rowntree Foundation, a charity that campaigns to end poverty, an additional 400,000 people are in poverty as a result of the freeze.[13] Other changes in working age benefits, with policies such as the two-child limit on child benefit, the introduction of Universal Credit and the switch from Disability Living Allowance to Personal Independence Payment, have also had a negative impact on the incomes of working age adults, including those with disabilities. While the triple lock may have increased the value of the pension relative to working age benefits, this should not be an argument for reducing the value of the pension. Let's not frame the debate as a choice between returning to pensioner poverty or ending working-age poverty. We can make other choices (or at least our elected politicians can) between tax cuts, such as raising the threshold at which higher rate taxes kick in or uprating the state pension *and* working age benefits to keep pace with rising inflation and cost of living.

It is vital that the state pension continues to provide a level of minimum income that maintains its value relative to average earnings. We cannot and should not return to the 1980s and 1990s when the value of the state pension fell. This is critical for future pensioners as much as it is for today's pensioners.

AT WHAT AGE SHOULD WE GET THE STATE PENSION?

The basic state pension, introduced in 1948 by the National Insurance Act 1945, was universal and provided a flat-rate amount to women from age 60 and men from age 65. Despite the huge increases in life expectancy described in chapter 1, the state pension age remained constant for decades. While the original decision to equalise state pension ages between men and women was taken in 1995, the first increase in the age of entitlement was not implemented until 2010, when women's pension age began to slowly increase to 65. Further legislation in 2011 proposed accelerating the implementation dates. Further increases are planned for men and women with the state pension age going up to 66 in 2020 and to 67 between 2026 and 2028 (this was originally going to be between 2034 and 2036, but the increase was brought forward).

The Pensions Act 2014 required there to be regular reviews of the state pension age (at least once every five years). The first independent review was conducted by John Cridland, former Director of the Confederation of British Industry and Chair of Transport for the North. His review examined data on projections of life expectancy and healthy life expectancy, modelled various options to understand the impact on 'affordability', as viewed by the Treasury, and took evidence from a wide range of organisations. He recommended that the state pension age should increase further to age 68 between 2037 and 2039, seven years earlier than the government's current timetable. At the time of writing the government has not legislated to implement these changes.

It seems logical that, as we are living longer, the state pension age needs to increase to keep pace with this. So are these proposed increases in state pension going to be sufficient to close the affordability gap? Is this the solution to the pensions crisis?

Simply raising the state pension age will, in the long run, reduce the proportion of our national wealth that we spend on the state pension by a small amount (estimates suggest Cridland's proposals would reduce state pension spending by about 0.3 percentage points over 50 years).[14] Increasing the state pension age gradually is unlikely to make a radical impact on affordability, so should the state pension age increase more dramatically? As life expectancy has risen (but the state pension age has not), the length of time we spend in retirement has also increased. When the state pension was first introduced in 1908 for 70-year-olds, the small proportion who reached this age could expect to be in receipt of an old age pension for just 6.6 years.[15] The principle underpinning current policy on state pension age is to support people to spend, on average, one third of their adult life in retirement. Should we be more radical and increase state pension age to reduce the amount of time we can expect to be retired to, say, a quarter or a fifth of our adult lives?

The problem with this approach to setting the state pension age is that it is based on average life expectancy. The problem with averages is that they mask huge variations. Dr John Beard, former Director of Ageing and Life Course at the World Health Organisation, expands on this: 'There are inherent inequities in pension systems based on chronological age. If you're better off, you will live for longer and therefore you will benefit from pensions for longer, while poorer people get less benefit and yet have a greater need for a financial backstop.' Many people in deprived communities experience ill health and disability on average 15 to 20 years earlier than people in wealthier communities, meaning more of them find it difficult to stay in work until state pension age. In the UK, disability-free life expectancy at birth is 62.7 for men and 61.9 for women, meaning the majority reach pensionable age with at least one disability.[16] This is a problem I look at in the chapters on health and work.

To this end, some groups have proposed that access to the state pension age should vary according to a person's circumstances. Suggestions have included: allowing long-term carers to access their pensions early; having different state pension ages geographically according to average life expectancy in that place; or allowing individuals earlier access based on their anticipated lifespan. Cridland rejected these proposals as complex and unworkable, while calling on government to mitigate the impact of raising the state pension age on those who would find it difficult to keep working. He recommended that some of these inequalities be tackled through the benefits system, rather than by changing the universal state pension age, in order to alleviate the impact on low-earners, carers and people in ill health.[17] In his report he proposes that those who are unable to work due to caring responsibilities or ill health should get access to Pension Credit a year earlier. He also proposes that older job seekers, those on Universal Credit and those who would qualify for the means-tested Pension Credit should not be penalised for taking part-time work. At present they would be expected to look for full-time work.

Adair Turner, former Chair of the Financial Conduct Authority and Chair of the Pensions Commission, which was set up under the Labour government in 2002 and whose second report was published in 2005, also recognised that raising the state pension age was going to disproportionately affect poorer people who are more likely to be in poor health and have a disability. Until 2010 there was unconditional access to Pension Credit at age 60 for men and women. Eligibility for Pension Credit has gone up in line with the state pension age for women, so no-one gets it early now. One of the ideas was to freeze the age of eligibility for the means-tested Pension Credit as the state pension age rises, so someone could apply for Pension Credit at 65 even if they would not get the state pension itself until, say, 67. This would allow someone on a lower income to receive pension income earlier than other people, removing them from the working age benefits system which requires people to either continue seeking full-time work or prove they have a disability or health issue that prevents them from working.

Inequalities mean that more radical changes are needed to ensure those who 'age' prematurely, and experience the onset of health and disability earlier, are supported to make the transition from paid work to retirement. The ideas proposed by Adair Turner and John Cridland could make a positive difference, but we need to be more radical still and changes are needed now, not when further increases in the state pension age are implemented. Given the size of the inequalities in healthy life expectancy between rich and poor, access to Pension Credit five years earlier than the state pension age for low earners, carers and people in poor health, would be better than just a year, as proposed in the Cridland Review. This would remove the poorest from having to navigate the systems of assessment in order to prove their eligibility for Employment and Support Allowance, and reduce unnecessary costs to the state of people having to go through work capability assessments. The Department for Work and Pensions currently spends around £7 billion per year on the main out-of-work benefits for people aged 50 to state pension age.[18] Changes could ensure that this delivers better outcomes for individuals than the current system.

At the moment, with Universal Credit, the benefit that replaces a number of others, including Housing Benefit and Jobseeker's Allowance, there is conditionality, meaning that people have to take full-time jobs if available (not part-time). This needs to be flexed for those in the years before state pension age so that they could take a part-time role without penalty. Similarly, the approach to Jobseeker's Allowance for those five years before state pension age could be adjusted to recognise that not all available jobs will be suitable given the location and physicality of the work, and that if people of these ages are able to find suitable work it may be part-time. Requirements to undertake job-related training and limits on the amount of caring and voluntary work someone is allowed to do without it impacting on their benefits also need to be more flexible. Older job seekers might be encouraged to learn other skills and do activities which make a worthwhile contribution outside paid work.

Most people, when they stop work and draw their pension, experience a reduction in their income. Ironically for those on the lowest wages or working age benefits, they are actually financially better off when they reach state pension age. The Institute for Fiscal Studies recently said that the benefits for low-income pensioners has diverged dramatically from that for people just below state pension age, with the poorest fifth of people in the five years after reaching state pension age being 70% better off than the poorest fifth in the years leading up to it.[19] Most benefits, including Employment and Support Allowance and Jobseeker's Allowance, provide a lower weekly income than the state pension. In 2019-2020, Employment and Support Allowance and Jobseeker's Allowance had a maximum weekly entitlement of £111.65. Those on Pension Credit can get access to other sources of income, such as Housing Benefit, Council Tax Reduction and the Warm Home Discount Scheme, as well as accessing universal age-related entitlements, for example, the Winter Fuel Payment.

A more radical solution would be to eliminate the age eligibility altogether. If we think of the state pension as a form of universal basic income for those over state pension age, then why not go the whole hog and create a genuinely universal basic income for people of all ages? That would be a huge improvement on Universal Credit. Like the living wage, there could be an independent commission to set a 'living income' for people in different circumstances, to reflect the higher costs of living with a disability, for example. This would remove many of the barriers to proving eligibility for out-of-work benefits, whether as a carer, parent or because you are sick or have a disability. It would change the relationship between work and other non-paid activity, and value equally the contributions of people of all ages. In order to make this progressive it would have to be funded by raising taxes on those with higher incomes (effectively taxing back the cost of this), while also making sure allowances and tax rates for those on low earnings made work pay.

Fundamentally, linking the entitlement to state pension to chronological age fails to recognise that ability to work has little to do with our age. Either fundamental changes to the benefits system are needed to address these inequalities or a more radical option of a universal basic income, which does not discriminate by age, needs to be considered. It is important not just to look at age in isolation from the other aspects of the state pension, so let's turn to other arguments about who should be entitled to it.

WHO SHOULD GET THE STATE PENSION?

Voluntary occupational pensions were originally designed as income protection for workers when they were no longer able to work due to their age. Eligibility was based on contributions. The original proposal for the 1948 basic state pension was that it should be fully funded, with an individual's contributions over their working life being sufficient to fund a basic pension income in future. However, there was an immediate need to fund pensions for the current older generation, so the scheme that was implemented was actually 'pay as you go'. This is still the case in the UK today – pensions are paid for out of taxation and National Insurance receipts levied on *today's* workers, despite the fact that some people believed that the National Insurance contributions they paid in the past – paying their stamp – was paid into a 'fund' for them to access when the time came.

Those retiring before April 2016 required 30 qualifying years to receive a full state pension. This resulted in those with interrupted working lives, particularly women and those with caring responsibilities, receiving a lower pension. For a long time, the system penalised women, who either relied on their husband's pension or a widow's pension. Only 36% of women aged 65 to 69 received the full state pension in 2014,[20] but reforms to pensions made in 2010 mean carers and those on adoption, paternity or maternity leave, as well as those entitled to child benefit or foster carer allowance, are able to claim contributory years. However, awareness of this has been low and people missed out on claiming these credits, although some are automatically credited now.

Since April 2016 and the introduction of the new state pension, someone has to have 35 qualifying years of contributions to get the full amount and a minimum of 10 qualifying years to get anything. There is a complex system of credits which enable some people, such as those on Jobseeker's Allowance, Universal Credit, Employment and Support Allowance, maternity pay and Carer's Allowance, to get credits automatically. For those who qualify, these credits are added to their insurance record and count as qualifying contributions for state pension entitlement. Pensions are also now calculated on an individual basis, so National Insurance contributions can no longer be shared or transferred between married couples.

Ultimately, we need to be clear on the objectives of the state pension. If it is to ensure a basic income for everyone of a certain age, then that raises a question about having a contributory principle at all. Making the pension truly universal could be done by making length of residency in the UK the basis, rather than number of years making National Insurance contributions. Adair Turner, in his 2005 Pensions Commission report, proposed that the pension should be made 'universal', with eligibility based on residence (i.e. how long you have lived in the UK) rather than contributory years, and 'individual' (i.e. no longer linked to your spouse's pension).[21] Such a simplification of the pension system would remove the need for people who are not active in the labour market to claim credits for non-contributory years and would also reduce the bureaucracy and stigma associated with applying for Pension Credit.

By far the most radical and unpopular of the options to make the state pension 'affordable' is to means test it. The original state pension in 1908 was means tested, but since 1948 the state pension has been universal in the sense that everyone who has contributed is eligible, regardless of income. What would be the impact of a return to means testing?

The reality is that nearly half of the population (49%) rely on the state pension for the majority of their income in later life.[22] According to the Department for Work and Pensions, in 2016-2017 on average the income of a household unit over 75 years old was made up of 54% from the state pension and benefits, 30% from private pensions, 5% from earnings and 8% from investments. The same statistics show that the poorest fifth of single pensioners get nearly 90% of their income from the state pension. Any changes would impact women particularly badly, with the average single female pensioner deriving 65% of their weekly income from the state pension and associated benefits, while these make up just less than half (49%) of weekly earnings for the average single male pensioner.[23] Any means-tested pension would still have to be paid out to a large proportion of the population who rely on it.

The importance of the state pension as a source of income also increases with age, as private pensions are exhausted, the purchasing power of pay-outs that are not inflation-linked reduces and the option to supplement income with paid work becomes more difficult. My father-in-law had a small occupational pension, but the value of this did not keep pace with inflation, so by the time he was 87, his pension could only buy 58% of what it could in 1995 when he retired. When he died, my mother-in-law only got half of the amount as a widow's pension, but the costs of running the house where she lives have only continued to rise.

The problem with means testing is that it requires a bureaucracy to run it and those who are just above the eligibility threshold are often worse off. There is also a risk that it will create disincentives to save at a time when, as we will see, there is a need to drastically increase savings rates, especially at lower levels of earnings. At the moment, whatever amount people are able to save into private pensions has no impact on how much state pension people get. In Australia pensions are means tested using a taper, which means that as wealth and assets increase the amount of pension reduces. If housing wealth were taken into account, this would penalise low-income pensioner home-owners, who would be forced to sell up – something that has proven very unpopular as a way of funding social care.

As we have seen, only 60% of pensioners who are eligible for the current means-tested Pension Credit actually claim it. This is lower than the proportion of eligible claimants who claim working age benefits, suggesting either: ignorance – they don't know about the benefit; complexity – the process of making a claim is difficult; or stigma – they are ashamed not to be financially self-reliant. Means testing pensions can appear to be progressive – why use limited public money to fund a universal pension when some people could afford to have a decent standard of living without it? However, the practicalities are likely to mean those who need it most would be hardest hit.

Affordability of pensions has been framed by the doom-mongers in such a way that it focuses only on how to *reduce* public spending on state pensions. A lot of debate, therefore, has focused on paying out less in state pensions to fewer people and for less time by raising the state pension age and abolishing the triple lock. This approach will not deliver good outcomes and there is a risk that the costs are simply passed on to the wider welfare system through things like means-tested Pension Credit, Housing Benefit and the like.

When I spoke to John Cridland, he argued that reforms to the state pension had dealt with many of the problems that had previously existed: the triple lock means that the value of the pension relative to average earnings has recovered; the introduction of credits for various benefits means more people are receiving the state pension; and credits for those with caring responsibilities mean women are not out of pocket as much as they were in previous generations. However, he felt there is more to do to address inequalities, particularly in the benefits system.

It is important that pension policy provides people with long-term certainty. Enshrining some clear principles about who is eligible, at what age and what will give more people confidence that they will be guaranteed a minimum income in old age, when they are no longer able to work, and will not be penalised for saving more or for working longer. The real question is how much we are willing to pay collectively to ensure that everyone has a decent income in old age or, at a minimum, to protect people from living out their old age in poverty.

Current generations have almost given up on the hope that the state will provide for them in retirement. In a 2012 survey by the Department for Work and Pensions on attitudes to pensions, 38% of respondents thought that there wouldn't be a state pension by the time they retired. This view was particularly pronounced in younger respondents.[24] For many people now and in the future, the state pension is likely to provide little more than a safety net to keep them out of poverty (even if the triple lock is maintained). Whatever additional income we want in old age we will have to save ourselves. This is where private pensions come in.

THE RISE OF PRIVATE SAVINGS

There has been an international push to reform public pensions, led by the World Bank, International Monetary Fund (IMF) and OECD. They are concerned about the large future liabilities that governments will have as a result of commitments and promises made under both state pension schemes and large public-sector pension schemes, such as that for NHS employees in the UK, and for civil servants and public workers in countries like Germany, France and Spain. Economists working in these global economic institutions believe future state pension liabilities will put too great a burden on public spending, act as a drag on economic growth and increase the size of public debt beyond levels deemed to be sustainable. In other words, the debt repayments would be higher than the country could afford to fund through taxation. In place of these public pensions, they have encouraged governments to expand private pensions, but as we will see, these are not without their problems.

The UK has reformed the public pension system far more radically than many other countries. The UK led the way on pension reforms in the 1980s, with major reforms to public pensions and a dramatic switch to private pensions. Other countries continue to have much larger liabilities, in part because their pay-outs are also linked to earnings, so they face an even bigger challenge of how to fund the pensions of a growing number of pensioners from a shrinking tax base. The box on page 60 illustrates the challenges facing Brazil, a country which is going through the age shift very rapidly, and which has a generous and unreformed public pension system.

In the UK, some public pension schemes have been privatised. Industries privatised during and after the Thatcher period, such as BT and British Coal, were also forced to take their liabilities with them. In other words, they remained responsible for funding the pensions of those workers to whom they had already made commitments, effectively switching the responsibility for paying the pensions from the state to the company. The majority of these schemes are protected by Crown Guarantees, which means that if the company were to collapse and be unable to meet their pension obligations, the government would be responsible for liabilities accrued prior to privatisation. The government also guaranteed the pensions of British Rail in 1994 and took on Royal Mail's liabilities in 2012 when it was part-privatised, so in the end taxpayers have underwritten the pensions to provide that guarantee.

Other reforms to public sector pensions have been introduced. For example, in many schemes the amount of pension shifted from a percentage of final salary to a career average salary, the

THE CHALLENGES OF PENSION REFORM IN BRAZIL

People over 65 currently make up less than 8% of Brazil's population, but the rate at which the population is predicted to age means there must be significant changes to the current system of work and retirement: a 300% increase in the number of older people is predicted, from 14 million in 2012 to 49 million in 2050.[25]

One of the biggest challenges Brazil faces is its expenditure on pensions. Public spending on pensions constituted 14% of GDP in 2019, despite the over 60s being only about 12% of the population. The generous pensions system in Brazil is largely responsible for the budget deficit, alongside other social security spending, with 73% of the federal primary spending budget committed to social security and assistance in 2019.[26] Although the state pension is linked to previous earnings, there is a strongly redistributive effect as pension increases are linked to minimum wage increases, so the least wealthy benefit most from the state pension. Reform has proven difficult, since pension rights are written into the 1988 constitution and thus would require an amendment. Between 1988 and 2013, life expectancy increased by nearly 13 years.[27]

There is currently no established retirement age and retirement is based on contributing years rather than a minimum age. If you were to start your career at 20, it would be possible to retire at 55 for men and 50 for women under the current rules. Although there is a somewhat shorter life expectancy than in other countries, this gap is not sufficiently wide to justify the retirement gap. OECD research has concluded that the existing pension system is financially unsustainable, especially given the rate at which Brazil is anticipated to age.[28] In late 2019, despite strong opposition from trade unions and other professional groups, President Jair Bolsonaro's government passed sweeping reforms which will increase the pension age and reduce entitlements.

age at which people could draw the pension increased (from 60 to 65 for both doctors and teachers, for example), and some schemes were closed to new entrants. The government predicts that expenditure on current pensioners in receipt of public sector pensions, currently 2% of GDP, will fall to 1.5% over the next 50 years, having peaked in the next decade, largely due to the impact of these reforms.[29] These pensions continue to be generous compared to private pensions and are unlikely to be dramatically reduced further. Public sector pension reform has been politically toxic – striking doctors and firefighters don't make for happy headlines. One of the most significant changes in (public and private) occupational pensions is the demise of defined benefit pension schemes.

THE DEMISE OF DEFINED BENEFIT PENSIONS

For much of the second half of the 20th century, workplace pensions provided another mechanism for people to save for old age. The majority of these schemes were what are called defined benefit schemes. The employer and employee both paid in a proportion of the wages to the scheme. In return, the employee would be guaranteed an income linked to their salary. The percentage would depend on the number of years that someone had been a member of the scheme. In the public sector these large schemes were funded through taxation. In private sector schemes the pension fund was either managed by the company itself or managed on behalf of the company by a private pension provider, or a trust-based scheme (where the employer appoints trustees to run the pension fund).

The shift from defined benefit (the scheme where the amount you receive is linked to your earnings) to defined contribution (where the amount you receive is linked to the amount you contribute, plus any interest gained through performance of the investments) has happened in both the public and the private sector. Between 1997 and 2015, membership of defined benefit pensions fell from 45.7% of the workforce to 28.3%. This gap was filled by defined contribution pensions, which rose from 8.7% to 18% of all workplace pensions in the same time frame.[30] Nearly 8 million people are still active members of defined benefit pension schemes, although in the private sector these have largely been closed to new entrants and replaced with defined contribution pensions, effectively shifting the risk from the company to the individual.[31]

Why did this shift happen? With defined benefit schemes the risk sits with the company. The combination of rising life expectancy (higher than had been predicted) together with falling investment returns meant that many of these schemes were under-funded relative to their liabilities – there wasn't enough money in the pot to meet all the pay-outs for current and future pensioners. In order to ensure the financial sustainability of these pension funds, companies have been faced with making large cash injections, as well as increasing contribution rates from current members. Pension regulations require independent valuation of these schemes (usually every three years) and recommendations are made about how much additional money needs to be put in to top up the pot. Many defined benefit pension schemes are struggling to meet these payments, with the Department for Work and Pensions estimating in 2016 that 90-95% of defined benefit pension schemes were in deficit.[32]

You can imagine that for businesses with their own pension funds these payments have been a drag affecting their ability to compete. New companies with no pension schemes are not burdened with the same financial obligations as long-established companies, for example, giving EasyJet an advantage over British Airways in the airline industry. Companies are having to take the money out of profits, reduce capital investment or reduce operating costs, for example, by keeping wages low. Resolution Foundation's Intergenerational Commission found that defined benefit deficit payments were directly lowering pay by between £1.4 billion and £2.2 billion a year.[33] In order to transfer this risk, occupational pension funds in the private sector have not only transferred the management of the pension funds, but are also transferring the assets and liabilities to large financial companies. For example, in 2018 Legal and General took on £4.4 billion of pension liabilities from British Airways, covering 22,000 people in their final salary scheme and 60% of the total assets in the pension fund. These so-called bulk annuity deals were predicted to be worth in excess of £30 billion in 2019 as higher interest rates and slowing life expectancy growth mean the funds are in a better financial position.[34]

Some of the companies with large pension liabilities have gone bankrupt, leaving current and future pensioners high and dry (as well as large numbers of people out of a job). Unfortunately, pension protections are weak. Even pensions covered by the Pension Protection Fund (PPF) are not guaranteed to be paid in their entirety should an organisation go into administration. After British Home Stores recently closed, people holding pension entitlements could either transfer their funds to a new scheme with similar but not equivalent benefits, take a lump sum if eligible, or remain in the current PPF-protected fund, retaining about 90% of the original value of their pensions.[35] The PPF, whose job it is to take on the liabilities of insolvent pension funds, has taken on a large number of schemes in the last few years. After construction company Carillion went bust in 2018, it did so with pension liabilities of more than £2.6 billion and 27,000 members in active receipt of final salary pensions. This is the biggest hit to the PPF since its inception.[36] These high-profile failures do not build confidence in private workplace pensions. Perhaps businesses should be required to insure their pension liabilities in case they go into administration?

Have private individual savings fared any better? Mis-selling scandals in the late 1980s and early 1990s undermined public trust in pensions. Members of occupational pension schemes were persuaded to switch to a personal pension often based on hugely inflated projections of investment returns. Fees were high and often lacked transparency. A significant number of those who were mis-sold pensions were members of public sector defined benefit schemes which would have paid them significant sums in retirement. The products they were sold were dependent on the performance of the stock market and, as a result, their pay-outs in retirement were much lower than predicted. Plans often tied people in so that on retirement they had to buy a particular product (usually an annuity which paid out a regular amount of income until death). The economic crisis in 2008 further undermined the role of private financial companies in pension provision. Data from the Department for Work and Pensions suggests that confidence levels in financial companies to both guarantee an income and to deliver sufficient income declined by more than 20 percentage points between 2006 and 2009.[37]

Although defined benefit schemes have almost entirely been replaced with defined contribution schemes, meeting the pension promises already made is a big challenge, including to public sector workers, which will continue to cost the state significant sums into the future. Companies are rapidly ridding themselves of current and future pension liabilities, the state is picking up the pieces when companies go bust and individual consumers have lost confidence in private pension providers. As a result, there are too few people saving and they are saving too little. And there are people who are not saving at all. So what solutions are currently being tried to solve this problem?

ARE CURRENT REFORMS WORKING?

There has been a raft of pension reforms in recent years to try and address some of the problems I've outlined. These include:

- the phased introduction of auto enrolment between 2012 and 2017, aimed at increasing the number of people saving by enrolling everyone in a workplace pension unless they opt out;
- pension freedoms introduced in 2015 aimed at increasing competition in the retirement products market by giving people more choices about how they use their retirement savings; and

- further changes are proposed, including the introduction of a pension dashboard to bring together information about different pension pots in one place.

Don't worry, I'm not about to offer you advice on making your own savings decisions, but I do want to assess whether these changes are going to be enough to enable more of us to be financially secure in later life or whether we need more radical alternatives.

MORE SAVERS

Simon, one of the thriving boomers I introduced earlier, is a retired engineer and was able to carefully manage his finances and put aside extra savings for about 10 years before he stopped working. Although he's retired, Simon occasionally does some contract work and might do more in the future.

Simon is perhaps a stereotypical wealthy boomer, but others approaching later life don't feel able to save money while they're working and, like Rachel, are juggling competing priorities and probably not saving enough.

One of the squeezed middle-aged, she has three part-time jobs and her husband works full time. However, their outgoings are high, with a mortgage and two sons at university. Although Rachel is saving into small pensions with her part-time jobs, and her husband is paying into two more, she feels financially unprepared for retirement and worries that she won't ever be able to retire entirely.

Many people think about these issues too late. For others life events happen and prevent them from saving or contributing to a pension. For many others there simply isn't the money to save when the bills are paid. So how can we increase the number of people saving and the amount they save? One solution that has already been adopted in the UK is auto enrolment.

These reforms were partly inspired by the fathers of 'nudge', Richard Thaler, winner of the Nobel Prize in Economics in 2017, and Professor Cass Sunstein of Harvard Law School, whose experiments and research showed it was possible to increase participation using 'defaults', such as making people opt out rather than opt in. Their ideas have been applied to a wide range of issues, including increasing the rates of organ donation. Automatic enrolment requires employers to enrol workers who were ordinarily resident in the UK, aged over 22 and earning more than £10,000 a year. The government's review of automatic enrolment showed a significant rise in the number of people contributing to a pension, from 42% of eligible employees in 2012 to 87% in 2018.[38]

Auto enrolment has helped more people to join a pension scheme, but it doesn't really do anything at the moment about people who are self-employed, where there is no incentive to save as there are no employer contributions. According to analysis of the Labour Force Survey by the Association of Independent Professionals and the Self-Employed, nearly one in three of those who are solo self-employed said they were not currently saving into a private/personal pension, and 30% of the self-employed over 50 have no private pension wealth at all (although many have retained occupational entitlements from earlier in their working lives).[39] While auto enrolment has increased the proportion of employees saving into a pension, there's been a reduction in the number of self-employed actively saving into a private pension, from 35% in 2007-2008 to 15% in 2017-2018.[40] Matthew Taylor, Chief Executive of the Royal Society of Arts, led a government review of self-employment in which he proposed auto-enrolling self-employed people and administering this through the self-assessment process. The government needs to consider whether to provide additional incentives, for example, by paying the equivalent of the employer contribution, to encourage more self-employed people to contribute to pensions or providing the equivalent incentive in the form of tax credits.

SAVING MORE

Making saving automatic, rather than a rational choice, has made people more likely to contribute, but are they saving enough?

Currently, the vast majority of people are not. While more than 50% of the population aged 65 and over have a private pension pot, on average this is small.[41] The majority of pension pots are below £20,000 in value. If a pot of this size were invested in a lifetime annuity – a financial product that guarantees a fixed sum each month or year for the rest of your life – it would only generate approximately £700 in income per annum.[42] The government suggests we need our pension income to be about two thirds of our final salary to maintain our lifestyle on retirement – this is what is called the replacement rate. However, this generally assumes that there will be no housing costs, because people own their homes and have paid off their mortgages. As we will see in the chapter on housing, in future there will be many more private renters, people who only own a portion of the equity in their home under shared ownership models or who have outstanding mortgage payments. If people have to continue to meet housing costs in retirement, they will need something closer to a 100% replacement rate. It is perhaps worth pausing to have a quick think about how much you would need to live comfortably in retirement (if you're not already retired) and what proportion of your wages you are saving now. I bet you're not saving enough.

We can try and help people have more realistic expectations about how much they might need to save to get a certain standard of living. Ready reckoners, like the one that the Pensions and Lifetime Savings Association has developed, are a useful rule of thumb for consumers, but how many people are likely to consult this and even if they do will they act on it? We can try engaging people earlier in thinking about their savings, but the evidence suggests that unless this is linked to a focus on wellbeing and what you want to do with the rest of your life, people won't engage. And those on low incomes have other more immediate priorities, are often managing debts, and are much less likely to plan and prepare for the future.

So how much is enough? Most of us haven't a clue how much we should be saving during our working lives if we want to enjoy a reasonable standard of living. And our living standards in old age are not only determined by the size of our pension and the income it provides, but also by other factors, such as: our health and ability to work; our life-time earnings, career breaks and caring responsibilities; our wealth and assets, accumulated or inherited; whether or not we own our home or have a mortgage or other debts; and whether we have family members to support us, either financially or by providing care or somewhere to live. There are also many choices. For example, do you intend to reach 'peak earnings' in your 50s and 60s then retire early or do you plan on a phased retirement, taking a part-time or less stressful job (that also pays less)? Do you want to blend taking a partial pension and topping this up with earnings? What is the best way to manage earnings and income over a lifetime, especially a longer life? And are you banking on your house being your pension? If so, what are the pitfalls of this? The options and trade-offs can be bewildering.

So how much would the median earner need to save as a proportion of their salary to achieve a 'modest' income of, say, £17,500 per annum? If the state pension continues to be uprated using the triple lock, as now, they would have to contribute 8.4% of their earnings each year from the age 22. If the state pension was only increased in line with earnings inflation, the same person would have to contribute 9.2%.[43] In reality, the average contribution rate for someone in an open defined contribution scheme is just 2.7% of their salary, far below the level needed to achieve a decent replacement rate. Those in defined benefit schemes save significantly more, at an average of 6.9%. However, this is still not enough.[44] And most of us won't consistently save from 22, particularly those who take career breaks and have other priorities on a limited income. In fact, the Department for Work and Pensions has estimated that 12 million people, making up nearly 40% of the working age population, are under-saving for retirement.[45] It's perhaps little surprise, then, that most of us only save when we are compelled to or when it is made automatic. (See the box on page 69 for a successful nudge experiment from the US.)

When they were first introduced, the auto enrolment contribution rates were very low: 1% of earnings for the employer and 1% for the employee, between 2012 and February 2018, when all employers needed to comply with the law. From April 2019 the rates have increased to 3% and 5% respectively for the employer and employee. There is a risk that, as contribution rates increase, more people will opt out. If this starts to happen, the government will have to consider whether to reduce the contribution levels, in the sure knowledge that people's savings will fall short, or make contributions compulsory, thus violating the principles of the nudge approach. It also doesn't leave people much choice about other priorities that they may have for saving, which is something I'll address as we look to the future below.

NUDGING PEOPLE TO SAVE MORE

The Save More Tomorrow is an American pension programme, which started as a project led by behavioural economists Richard Thaler and Shlomo Benartzi in Chicago. The initial research demonstrated the impact of behavioural interventions for pension savings. The programme saw employees enrolled into a workplace pension scheme, which initially required them to save only small amounts, while committing to increasing their contributions in the future. As their salary increased, their contributions were automatically increased for them.

This approach removes the need for action to increase contributions and can fill the gap between how much people are saving and how much they can, and want to, save. Of the initial group, most remained in the programme up to the maximum of four pay rises. Average savings rates of those employees in the plan rose from 3.5% before they received advice to 13.6% after the fourth pay rise.[46]

The success of the study led to the widespread adoption of 'nudge' techniques by US pension schemes, with automatic opt-ins and contribution rises. In 2006, a federal law encouraged companies to adopt the principles of the scheme, which is estimated to have increased the saving rates of millions of Americans.

Women are particularly at risk of not having adequate pensions and, due to the structure of pensions, are more likely than men to experience poverty and financial problems in later life, despite higher levels of labour participation by women at older ages. Many older women, in particular, find themselves financially insecure; without a full state pension (due to lack of contributory years) and with only a very modest personal pension, if any. Women are penalised at every turn, with lower lifetime earnings because of part-time work, the gender pay gap, and interrupting their work to care for children and older relatives. They are unlikely to get access to the full amount of their husbands' pension if they divorce and, if widowed, have a much-reduced income compared to the one they enjoyed when their husbands were alive. Women who have spent the majority of their careers in part-time work are no better off in retirement than women who have never been in paid work.[47] There is also a compounding of disadvantages for some women, for example, women who are divorced, identify as LGBTQ or are from a Black and Minority Ethnic (BAME) background, meaning they are much less likely to be able to accumulate adequate resources for their later lives.[48]

There are many women in Kate's position. One of the 'downbeat boomers' from the Later Life Study, Kate, is 63 and married with two older daughters, one of whom has moved back to live with them after her relationship broke up, while the other has recently had a baby. Kate worries about having enough money in the future, for home repairs or if one her daughters needs financial help. When it comes to planning for her own later life, Kate is relying on her husband, who is ten years younger than her, and the plans he has made for their later life. This means that if Kate and her husband were to split, she does not have a back-up plan for financing her later life. It is important that women are encouraged to save more, but also that pension flexibilities allow working spouses and partners to contribute to their partner's and spouse's pensions, during a career break for example, and that calculations regarding pension values are made as part of divorce settlements.

The number of people saving into private pensions is rising, thanks in part to auto enrolment, but many people are not saving at levels that will deliver adequate income in retirement. Action is needed to boost savings further, although this will be difficult given competing pressures on household income, and a significant increase in the savings rate for auto enrolment is likely to push more people to opt out. Going beyond 'nudge' and making contributions to private schemes compulsory risks distorting priorities and fails to recognise other ways in which people save.

REDUCING COMPLEXITY

Making savings decisions is hard, as I discovered when I tried out one of the many online pension calculators. I'd just received my pension statement from my previous employer, so I had the information to hand. Here's what I found out.

For starters, it suggested I would need to work until I'm 70. Given the research that being in fulfilling work in later life can have positive benefits, this did not worry me too much. Both my parents-in-law had worked well into their 70s, partly motivated by financial necessity, but it also kept them active and they clearly enjoyed the social aspects of work.

Second, the tool suggested how much I should be saving to my pension each month. The current state of the financial markets and the prospect of negative interest rates meant the level of growth I could expect on any savings were very uncertain. I pride myself on being reasonably numerate and yet these uncertainties left me unsure whether I am doing the right thing.

The tool also highlighted the consequences of not having saved enough – a period of later life in which I would have to live off the state pension and a modest income from the small defined benefit pension schemes I had contributed to early in my career. What the tool did not do was give me a realistic view of what quality of life the money would buy so far in the future. If I look back 50 years, standards of living and the cost of living have changed beyond recognition. How will they look in 50 years? The information needs to make it much clearer for everyone, whether on low incomes or higher incomes, the lifestyle their retirement income could buy.

People generally find pensions bewildering. Incredibly, even those working in the pensions system find it hard to keep track of their investments. Andy Briggs, who was chief executive officer for UK insurance at Aviva, one of the largest insurers in the UK, confessed that he found it personally challenging to keep track of what his expected retirement income might be. People simply don't know what pensions they have and what income they might generate. Pension funds now issue an annual statement letter which sets out how much the pension is worth if you took it as a lump sum today and how much money you would receive when you retire (with some guarantee if it's a defined benefit pension but with a great deal of uncertainty if it's a defined contribution scheme). On average, people will have 11 jobs in their working lives, meaning they could have 11 different pensions when they retire.[49] Under auto enrolment, every time someone moves jobs they are usually enrolled in the scheme selected by the employer. Keeping track of these multiple schemes is challenging.

In 2016, the government proposed the idea of a pensions dashboard, which would bring together information in one place. The complexity of drawing together information from more than 40,000 pension schemes means there are now likely to be multiple commercial and non-commercial dashboards.[50] The government is working with the Money and Pensions Service (MaPS) and others in the sector to implement this. If properly implemented, this could have addressed some of the problems of keeping track of different pension pots, enabling people to more easily consolidate and move funds between pension pots and get better returns on their savings. However, this will only ever be the case for the most active consumers. Most people, particularly under auto enrolment, are not at all engaged with their pension savings.

Consumer engagement research undertaken by pensions charity, the Pensions Policy Institute, suggested that there are a number of reasons why people don't engage with their pensions. This included people who were sceptical about putting their trust in pension providers, as well as those who are starting out in their careers and are focused on other financial priorities.[51] With changes in the labour market it's even less likely that people will stay with the same company or indeed have only one employer. Do we need a pension that follows the person around? Employers would have to pay into multiple pots, in the same way as they currently pay wages into multiple bank accounts. It would also mean people choosing their own pension savings account rather than having one chosen for them by their employer, but this, too, could engage them earlier in the process.

ENABLING INFORMED CHOICE

In 2005, the government introduced pension reforms promoting 'freedom and choice'. The idea was to give people with a defined contribution pension more options on retirement (well, actually from age 55!). They no longer have to purchase an annuity (a product which guarantees a regular payment) and can instead leave the money where it is, get an adjustable income (called a flexi drawdown), take the cash in chunks, or cash in the whole pot (up to 25% tax free) or any combination of these options. Confused?

While these pension freedoms addressed one market failure, the mis-selling of pensions, it has created other problems. A review by the Financial Conduct Authority, the financial services regulator, in 2017 found that many consumers were drawing down their savings, rather than purchasing annuities as they had before. This means they have no guarantee of income and could exhaust their savings. It also found that over half of the defined contribution pension pots that had been accessed had been fully withdrawn. However, the majority were small in value with 90% under £30,000 and 60% under £10,000.[52] The fact that the freedoms kick in at age 55 also sends a signal that this is an acceptable age to retire and provides a disincentive to keep working longer, which could lead people to exhaust their savings if they underestimate how long they will live.

While these are important and complex decisions, the majority of people are taking them without advice, and many people take them without a good understanding of the choices and trade-offs. Research has suggested that about a third of people who began to withdraw the savings in their pension pot since 2015 did so without taking financial advice.[53] And there is good evidence that financial advice makes a difference in the pension options people choose. Nearly all (94%) who accessed their pension pots without taking financial advice took the drawdown option offered by their pension provider, compared to just over a third (35%) of those who took financial advice.[54] The cost of financial advice means that it is generally too expensive for the majority of people with only modest pension savings. To support people in making these decisions, PensionWise was set up by the government in 2015 to provide free, impartial guidance. This has just been merged into a new organisation with the catchy title of the Single Financial Guidance Body (aka the Money and Pensions Service).

So how will the provision of advice need to change to support better decisions? How does information need to be framed to enable better choices? Or should we return to a system where there are fewer choices and more compulsion or defaults? Experiments with automated advice using artificial intelligence and chatbots hold out the possibility of making advice more widely available, but it is likely that there will still need to be some human input into decision-making for a while yet. Until advice is more widely available and affordable it would be difficult to require people to take advice before accessing their savings. An alternative would be to set up some default products, including an annuity, which would simplify the choices people face.

The way that information is presented also doesn't help people make good decisions. We know from decision science that we value large sums in the present more than smaller sums in the future, so when defined contribution pension schemes send out an annual statement saying that the person is eligible to take a guaranteed (usually large) lump sum immediately, this can look more attractive than the promise of a regular sum for life (especially given that most people underestimate how long they will live), although the cumulative sum is likely to be much larger. The providers of pension information and guidance need to experiment with different ways of framing information and test the impact this has on people's decision-making.

Phillip Brown, formerly of the Financial Services Authority and now Managing Director at First 4 Knowledge, is quite clear that pension providers need to change the way they present information to customers: 'When you take out a pension, no-one says to you "You've done an amazing thing today to start securing your future." Instead what you get is a massive welcome pack with impenetrable language that talks to you about the contributions you're making and gives you policy numbers and schedules. You'll probably put it in a box somewhere or, in the worst-case scenario, you might throw it all away … The moment a company issues a glossary with their documents, they've completely failed in their objective of communicating with the customer. It horrifies me every time I see it.'

In practice, most financial advice is also limited to pensions and is often unable to provide a rounded view of all the things we want in life (such as studying or moving house) and the range of ways we might achieve this (such as buying a second property or working part-time). Of course, not all our savings or wealth are in the form of pensions either. In fact, an increasing share of wealth assets among people at older ages is made up of property wealth, due to the increases in housing equity and the numbers of people who own more than one property.

We also need to think more holistically about different savings options, and when and how much to access given our expectations about how long we will live (which, as we have seen, most people underestimate), how long we will work and how healthy we expect to be. We need help to join up the conversation about pensions, not only with considerations about housing wealth and other savings, but other aspects of our lives which will have financial implications, including support for other family members and the costs of care. John Cridland, author of the independent review into state pension age changes, recommended the idea of a mid-life MOT (see Legal and General mid-life MOT box on page 105) to support people to review health, finances and work. Several financial service providers have started to pilot these as a way of engaging customers. They're aimed at employees in 'mid-life', to help them understand what they can do to prepare for retirement. Often this involves a person visualising their later life and what kind of income they want, how they want to spend their time, and what steps they can take to build for that future now. In early 2019, the government launched a mid-life MOT website signposting people to guidance about preparing for retirement. They are also looking at new ways to engage people ahead of retirement with so-called 'wake up' packs.

If the reforms introduced as part of increasing freedom and choice are to be retained, then the regulatory rules also need to change to make impartial advice more widely available and accessible to everyone – in practice, it is mainly those with modest pension pots who are not engaging with financial advisors, according to research. There need to be more defaults, so that the many people who don't take advice are protected from making poor choices. The age at which these freedoms kick in needs to be much later than 55 and linked to life expectancy in the way that the state pension age is. Other behavioural techniques and ways of framing information that help people to plan, save and then manage their savings need to be trialled. These are all immediate changes that are needed to make the current system work better. Given how poorly we estimate our life expectancy and that we value certainty in the present over the uncertainty of a gain in the future, there is a real risk we will make poor decisions that will ultimately mean we run out of money and have to drastically reduce our living standards in old age. But what about future generations? What further changes are needed to enable them to plan ahead and secure a decent standard of living in old age?

LOOKING TO THE FUTURE

We have created a current system which is predicated on the three-stage life of education, work and retirement, described in the popular book, *The 100-Year Life,* by Lynda Gratton and Andrew Scott, both London Business School academics. We get our education when we are young, we then work to try and earn as much as possible (save what we can and avoid burning out), then retire and live off the savings we have managed to put away.[55] In the future this pattern will look very different. As we will see in the chapter on work, retirement may become a thing of the past. Perhaps the concept of a pension is also no longer useful. Instead, we need new financial products and incentives which enable us to smooth our income over the life course.

Millennials are spending longer in education, starting careers later and having families later.[56] According to Gratton and Scott, younger generations are also doing more 'exploring' – trying out different things before settling into a more permanent job and having more career breaks than older cohorts. They may have more debt, take out a mortgage later, if at all, and take longer to pay it off, and spend a greater proportion of their income on housing. Lack of wage growth and pay progression might also mean few people ever reach an earnings peak, but they may have more peaks and troughs as they take on a variety of roles and have multiple careers.

We will need to save at different times in our lives to fund the periods when we are not working, either because we are parenting, training, caring or refuelling. Financial services have not yet responded to the prospect of the 100-year life. We need the products to change, as well as the regulations and tax regime which govern this. At the moment the state and incentives around saving are all geared towards saving for retirement during a peak earning period in mid-life. We need financial services products which recognise the change in earning patterns being demonstrated by younger cohorts and which allow us to smooth income over the life course by saving flexibly when we are earning for the times when we are not earning. Perhaps we each need a personal wealth pot, for example, which can combine pensions savings including contributions from employers with our personal savings and from which we can take when we need to for different life events, rather than accessing it all in one go in retirement.

As long as people are doing some kind of long-term saving, this should be rewarded and encouraged. There needs to be a strong incentive to save and to leave what we have saved there for as long as possible, to counter our tendency to want to spend it and spend it now. The Lifetime ISA, which was launched by the then Chancellor George Osborne in 2016, was designed to do this, providing an additional tax-free subsidy. If the money is withdrawn, other than for buying a house or to fund retirement after age 55, this additional subsidy is lost.

Currently different types of savings and products have different tax treatments. and this adds to an already confusing picture for the consumer, so it is important that wealth, whether in property, pension savings or other savings, has the same tax treatment. Phillip Brown, the pensions expert I spoke to, highlighted the following problem: 'When I plan for my retirement, I don't just think about my pension. I think about the property I live in – I might be thinking about downsizing or moving to some sort of sheltered accommodation or releasing that asset. I might have things like individual savings accounts, cash savings. All of those things need considering, because your retirement is more than just this individual product. What the regulator, Treasury and HMRC need to think about is why do we put all these monies into different tax wrappers? I would contend that nobody gets up in the morning choosing to buy a specific tax wrapper.'

Even if people work for much longer in order to build up private savings, if they are going to save a lot more, they may have to be prepared to accept a lower standard of living throughout life. Instead of imagining that as we get older we earn more and can therefore spend more, we may need to reset expectations so that as we earn more we don't spend more but save more. This would mean decoupling living standards from fluctuations in income over the life course. This would mean a radical rethink of the rule of thumb that we need two-thirds of our salary as a replacement to maintain our living standard in retirement. It is vital that advice and guidance on how much to save is linked to choices and trade-offs about both current and future living standards, giving people a realistic view of whether they are 'on track' to (at least) maintain their current standard of living in retirement. Many people now bank online and get feedback on their spending patterns. It would be easy to use this data to 'nudge' people to save more for the future.

We also need to reset expectations that every generation will enjoy better living standards than the last. The current debate on living standards suggests that every generation has the right to be more prosperous than the one before, and this is the mark of a progressive and successful society. The Resolution Foundation's work around intergenerational injustice is all framed around the principle that each generation should have it better than the last. Politically, how do you get people to accept this change in living standards? Currently it's seen as a failure. Having it better is not just about consuming more. Let's stop measuring progress by how much wealth people have accumulated. Can we reframe progress as some have suggested and measure wellbeing or life satisfaction rather than income and wealth? We are already seeing a less consumerist and consumption-oriented trend emerge, mainly for environmental reasons. Matthew Taylor, Chief Executive of the RSA, agrees: 'Society as a whole needs to get this wisdom that quality of life involves family, community, learning and those kinds of things ... we need a post-materialistic term. It has started to happen in some ways because of climate change, for example.' We need a new intergenerational method for measuring progress that does not simply focus on whether the next generation are richer than the one before.

The doom-mongers argue the state pension is unaffordable and search for policy solutions to reduce how much we spend.

These include abolishing the triple lock, increasing state pension age further and faster, and reducing eligibility by introducing means testing. I would argue this is the wrong goal. The aim should be to ensure people are financially secure in later life. Yes, spending on state pensions is set to go up as the number of people of pensionable age increases, but the amount is quite predictable and even maintaining the triple lock does not pose a high risk to public finances. However, if we are going to enable more people to be financially secure in later life, we're going to have to have as the foundation a decent state pension.

The state pension will remain a vital source of income for people in later life in future. Indeed, perhaps even more so, given the disappearance of employer pension schemes with defined benefits, the high costs of housing, and the lack of wage growth and progression that some predict is here to stay. We should be talking about making it truly universal – available to everyone based on residence not contributions. This would go a long way to preventing the shocking gender inequalities we see today repeating themselves for generations to come.

If inequalities in healthy life expectancy continue to increase, then there must be action to ensure those whose health prevents them from working up to state pension age are not subject to financial hardship. Smoothing the transition from working age benefits to the state pension must be a priority for government and will require reform to the benefits system. Giving those on low incomes early access to Pension Credit could go some way to achieving this.

Currently the value of the state pension does little more than keep people out of poverty – and even then, it doesn't do so for everyone. We need to accept that if we want people in later life to be financially secure (or at a minimum not to live in poverty) then the cost of the state pension is a price we have to pay for longevity. Instead of debating whether to abolish the triple lock, we should be debating how to guarantee a decent standard of living for everyone into old age. An independent commission should be set up to define the value of a 'living pension' that would afford people a decent living standard in old age. This would not only guide policy on setting the value of the state pension, but help inform people about whether they are on target to save enough to top up this amount.

The UK has led the way on privatising pensions and yet the widespread insolvency of private occupational pension schemes, the transfer of these liabilities to large financial services companies and the fact that the state picks up the pension liabilities when a company goes bust suggest a reliance on private pensions is not going to deliver financial security for people in the changing labour market and with competing priorities.

While auto enrolment has increased the numbers of people saving and the amount being saved, at the end of the day these types of pensions (defined contribution schemes) shift all the risk to an individual. We build up an individual pot of money to invest with the hope that it will generate some sort of income for us in retirement. It seems unlikely that there will be a shift back towards occupational pensions (with defined benefits) any time soon. Other types of schemes, like the collective defined contribution pensions which exist in the Netherlands and Canada and are being considered for introduction in the UK, could offer an alternative. These pensions allow people to pool their contributions together and get a better investment return (over the long term) and lower fees.[57]

However, changes in home ownership and working patterns mean a total rethink of pensions is needed. People will want much more flexibility about how they accumulate savings and assets over a lifetime, and how and when they draw on them, for example, to buy a stake in a property or to retrain in order to work for longer. Financial services are stuck in an outdated model of the three-stage life. It is clear that the government will have to play an active role in creating a regulatory framework that encourages saving, ensures that everyone has access to affordable and impartial information and advice to manage their money at every stage of life, not just those who have a large pot on retirement, and that those providing the products are encouraged to innovate and respond to the needs of future, as well as current, retirees.

Even if people save privately towards a pension for most of their working life, it's unlikely to provide people with sufficient money to spend a third of their life in retirement. Whatever changes are made to both the state or private pensions, the fact is that if we want financial security in later life we will need to work longer. In the next chapter I'll look at what needs to change to support people to remain in work for longer.

4

The world of work

'We have a choice: a society where work becomes ever more dominant even as it becomes ever more precarious, where some work until they drop and others are demonised for being unable to work; or a society where we can realise our full potential in every sense, with more time for leisure, for love, for each other. I choose the latter. We should be striving to work less, not toiling until we drop.'

Owen Jones, *The Guardian* (March 2016)[1]

There is a worry that the lack of pension provision from the state and the inadequacy of private pensions will mean that many more of us will have to work for longer. The days of a long retirement spent on the golf course are over – if they ever existed. And yet if more older people stay in work, will this mean fewer jobs for the young? Shouldn't older people make way for younger workers? Older workers are accused of 'desk-blocking new talent.'[2] Is there a risk that an ageing workforce is less productive and will further stagnate the economy?

The reality is that there simply aren't enough young people entering the labour market to replace the numbers of older workers leaving. In 2018, UK job vacancies and numbers in work both hit record highs[3], adding to the pressure on employers to find and retain skilled staff. Growing skills and workforce shortages mean that businesses are competing for a shrinking pool of talent. The rate at which people are leaving the labour market is also accelerating as the baby boomers reach state pension age. It is a business imperative to retain older workers. So how does the world of work need to change to enable people to work for longer and at older ages?

Furthermore, rather than seeing these older workers as being a drag on productivity, we should be concerned about the productivity threat of a large proportion of people between 50 and state pension age who are not working. For some it's a choice – they are lucky enough to have savings or a pension which allows them to take early retirement. Others want to work, but don't, because of redundancy, ill health, disability or caring responsibilities. Finding more effective ways of supporting these people back into work would produce a huge economic dividend, as well as major benefits to their wellbeing and financial security. How does employment support need to change and what other issues need to be addressed if we are to close this economic activity gap? What could help these people, who often face multiple challenges, to return to work?

Work is less secure than it was and there are signs that lack of progression means people get trapped in low-pay, low-skilled jobs. How will this impact on the ability of younger generations to sustain a longer working life and their financial situation in later life?

I'll start by looking at how the face of the workforce is changing. I'll then consider the implications for employers and some of the actions they can take to support people to remain in work for longer. Finally, I'll look at the changing nature of work and why the quality of our jobs matters, too.

WHY BUSINESS NEEDS PEOPLE TO WORK LONGER

The workforce is increasingly an older workforce. Nearly one in three workers in the UK are aged 50 and over[4] and this is set to grow over the next decade. Aviva analysis of Office of National Statistics labour market statistics estimates the average age of a UK worker is now 41 years and 6 months – up from 38 years and 5 months in 1992.[5]

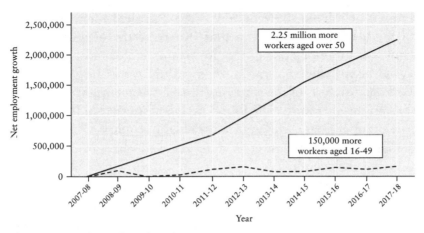

Change in numbers of workers by age group 2007-2008 to 2017-2018.
Source: *Annual Population Survey*, 2007-2008 to 2017-2018.

The graph above shows the change in the number of workers at different ages since 2007-2008. While there has been very little growth in the number of workers aged 16 to 49, there has been an increase of nearly 2.25 million workers aged over 50.

Some sectors have a higher proportion of older workers than others. Half of agricultural workers are over 50, with a further quarter over the age of 60. While 36% of workers in health and social care are over 50, only about 11% are over 60. There is a similar issue in the education sector. While 37% of teachers are over 50, many teachers retire before the age of 60, so only 12% are over 60.[6] As these people 'retire' or exit the labour market they leave a significant gap which is hard to fill given the numbers of young people coming into the labour market and levels of migration. For example, the Royal College of General Practitioners estimates that as many as 762 practices across the UK could close by 2023, because they rely on a workforce where three-quarters of GPs are aged over 55 and therefore able, and possibly even encouraged by the tax system, to retire and draw their pension.[7]

Are these older workers 'desk-blocking' – preventing younger workers from getting jobs? First, this assumes there are a fixed number of jobs in the economy – the so-called lump of labour fallacy – which would mean that if there were a higher rate of employment among one group, for example older workers, there would be a lower rate for another group, for example younger workers. Analysis of the relationships between employment rates at different ages in the UK found no evidence that older workers crowd out younger workers from the labour market.[8] The reality is that the labour market is dynamic and changes are closely linked to the economy.

International comparisons have shown that countries which have a higher proportion of older workers also have more younger workers, suggesting that jobs growth benefits all ages.[9] However, analysis of recent recessions suggests that increases in unemployment (even if relatively modest) were felt by those on low incomes, and increases were roughly twice as much for the younger age groups and those with fewer qualifications than for older workers and those with higher levels of qualifications. As we will see, this might be because changes in the labour market mean more people at younger ages are working in 'flexible' and less secure jobs or face redundancy simply because they are 'last in'.[10] The key to addressing this is not to encourage older workers to 'make way' for younger workers, but to return to economic growth (something that looks quite unlikely just now!) and to improve labour conditions so there are more good quality jobs that offer security and progression.

The reality is that the age shift in the population we are experiencing means those born during the 1960s baby boom will be leaving the labour market over the next 20 years. These workers are not easily going to be replaced. Why can't businesses simply hire and train more younger workers to replace those who are retiring? The answer: there simply aren't enough of them. Even if every young person was able to get a job, there would still be a labour and skills shortage. Between 2012 and 2022, if current trends continue, 12.5 million people will retire and a further 2 million new jobs will be created, but only 7 million young people will enter the workforce. This leaves a gap of 7.5 million jobs.[11]

Some other countries are worse off than the UK and face more severe labour shortages due to a rapidly ageing population, very low birth rates and, for example, in Japan, stricter immigration controls (see box below).

JAPAN'S LABOUR SHORTAGES

Japan already has higher rates of employment among people over pension age than many other countries. Despite many companies, including public sector organisations, having a mandatory retirement age of 60, nearly a quarter (23.5%) of people over 65 in Japan are economically active, compared to only 10.2% in the UK, but this is usually at a significantly lower wage than they would have received pre-retirement.[12] The state pension can currently be claimed between 60 and 70 years old (with the majority claiming at 65), but many people stay in work during and beyond their 60s. While just under 80% of large Japanese companies still had a mandatory retirement age of 60 in 2017, employment rates for older workers have risen. Since raising the retirement age would have significant wage implications due to the link between age and seniority, many companies have instead chosen to re-hire employees retiring at 60 in low-paid and low-productivity jobs until they claim their state pension at 65.[13] Despite this, Japan faces its biggest labour shortage in 40 years. Immigration remains a controversial public issue and non-Japanese workers constitute less than 1.5% of the workforce, compared to more than 5% in most developed economies, including nearly 10% of the UK workforce.[14]

Economic deals with the Philippines and Vietnam designed to help alleviate the 300,000 long-term care worker shortage Japan will face in the next 10 years has not resulted in anything like the numbers needed, as immigrant workers must be highly qualified and meet high Japanese language requirements. In response the Japanese government is looking to increase immigration by issuing five-year visas in specific industries, such as elderly care, agriculture and construction.

These proposals would relax Japanese language requirements, but workers would have to leave after five years and would not be permitted to bring family.

An alternative to immigration is the use of robotics. Shimizu, a construction company, tried out robots to help alleviate the labour shortage in construction. However, they could only use them at night due to health and safety concerns, and the robots were only able to do 1% of the work.[15] The government has also recently announced plans to address the shortage of some health care workers by building 10 'AI hospitals' by late 2022. These will use artificial intelligence to analyse test results and perform other tasks.

As the government imposes tighter immigration controls and the free movement of labour is restricted, as a result of the UK leaving the European Union, this will, in turn, increase the competition for skilled labour in the UK. It will therefore be vital for employers to retain older workers.

The loss of talent and knowledge as older workers exit work early is a silent brain drain that needs to be stemmed if UK Plc is going to have a prosperous future. Before we look at what needs to change to address this issue, let's look at when people currently stop work and why.

WHEN AND WHY DO PEOPLE RETIRE?

Nearly half (42%) of British adults say that they're looking forward to giving up work in the future.[16] There are a wide range of factors that will influence the age someone leaves work and whether this is something they chose to do (voluntary) or something that happens to them (involuntary).

Between 2006 and 2011 the default retirement age in the UK was 65. The introduction of a default retirement age was initially billed as a progressive move, as it meant companies could not force workers to retire *before* 65. However, Help the Aged and Age Concern (now Age UK) campaigned vocally against it, taking the government to the European Court of Justice in 2008. The European Union court ruled that a default retirement age was legal if it was for a legitimate aim linked to social or employment policy. The following year, however, the UK High Court judged that the government could not objectively justify such a policy. Subsequently, there was a stronger political appetite for changing the law and the abolition of the default retirement age was written into the Coalition Manifesto in 2010 and garnered particularly strong support in the House of Lords, where more than half of eligible members are over 70.[17] It was officially abolished in 2011.

The Equality Act 2010 introduced age as a protected characteristic, which means someone cannot be treated unfairly on the basis of their age (or how old they are understood to be). In the workplace this means an employer must not assume an employee is retiring, suggest they retire or try to force them to retire; to do so could be judged to be discriminatory. Consequently, most people should have a choice about when they want to retire. The reality is rather different.

First, some companies still require people to retire. Despite the fact that this was passed into law in 2011, both Oxford and Cambridge universities require certain high-ranking academics to retire at 68 and 67, respectively. A few other leading universities also still have retirement ages. They are able to 'objectively' justify this exemption in order to maintain their world-leading reputations and diversify their workforces.[18] Other professions in which you must retire at a certain age include the army, police, fire service, air-traffic control and the judiciary. Employers can lawfully require a retirement age if they can prove that it is objectively necessary. This Employer Justified Retirement Age has been used occasionally when a company sets a mandatory retirement age below state pension age. Often this is due to the physical or mental strain of the job, such as for an ambulance worker. However, there are a wide range of other jobs where, because the employment relationship is not clear or where the person is not technically an employee, such as a partner in a law firm or at one of the large consultancy firms, people can still be required to retire at a particular age.

Second, the incentives associated with some defined benefit pension schemes encourage people to retire early. For example, many public sector pension schemes pay out at 60 with the option of retiring earlier either on the same amount, if additional contributions have been made, or on a reduced amount. Some of those who are currently retiring are eligible for final salary pensions, which provides a disincentive to work part-time or take a lower level role as part of a gradual retirement. Some organisations made it difficult to draw a pension and return to work. The NHS has changed this and is now encouraging people to 'retire and return'. Staff can supplement their pension or delay drawing their pension until a later date while they continue to work. Other recent changes mean pension contributions in excess of an annual limit and lifetime allowance are subject to taxes. This has resulted in well-paid public sector workers, in particular doctors, retiring early to avoid paying these taxes or refusing to work additional hours or going part-time to avoid pushing their pensions contributions above the annual tax-free amount. Given the NHS has critical workforce shortages, the loss of these skilled and experienced doctors is a huge problem and the government is urgently looking to review these rules.

The third reason retirement may not be a choice is that redundancy can turn into early retirement. In 2015-2016, more than 10% of people aged 50-64 who reported themselves retired had left their last job due to redundancy or dismissal.[19] When there are restructuring and redundancies in organisations, older workers may be encouraged (actively or unconsciously) to take voluntary redundancy. They are often on higher salaries and entitled to higher redundancy packages due to length of service. Age discrimination also can work the other way, with companies making those who have more recently joined the firm redundant. This would disproportionately affect younger workers. The key is that there needs to be a justifiable business reason. Older workers who are made redundant have a much lower chance of returning to work, as we will see.

The whole decision about when to retire is not something that is openly discussed either. Part of the challenge is that retirement has become a taboo for both managers and workers. HR managers continue to express concern about how to handle conversations about retirement, with one qualitative study suggesting that managers felt reluctant to bring the subject of retirement up at all, believing that they will be open to accusations of age bias if they ask an older worker about their plans.[20] The Advisory, Conciliation and Arbitration Service (ACAS), an industrial relations organisation, has suggested that this conversation should be handled carefully, with all employees asked their plans for the short, medium and long term, to avoid the impression of targeting a specific worker of a certain age.[21] Career conversations should be the norm throughout someone's working life and so asking about future plans can open up conversations about whether someone is thinking about stopping work.

Even with the removal of the default retirement age and the option to defer taking the state pension, about one in four retired people in the Later Life Study said they'd retired simply due to reaching state pension age. In fact, the majority of women report that they retired because they reached state pension age. As the state pension age for women has risen, there has been an increase in the proportion of women remaining in work: between 2010 and 2017 the percentage of women aged 50-64 in work increased from 60% to 68%. Among women over 65 the increase was more modest, from 6% to 8%.[22] For men, involuntarily retirement, i.e. due to poor health or redundancy, is the most common reason. Among those who had worked in lower skilled manual jobs, 16% said the onset of ill health and disability was the main reason for retiring.[23]

Some people choose to work beyond state pension age. Professionals and those with higher levels of education are more likely to do so, whereas manual workers and those with lower levels of education are more likely to stop work at or before state pension age. A recent study found that 25% of those who retire return to work within five years. More research needs to be done on the concept of the 'unretired', but the evidence suggests that men, those with higher qualifications and those in better health are all more likely to return to work after retiring. However, the same study found that it is more difficult for disadvantaged older people to return to work, restricting their ability to supplement retirement income.[24]

We don't know why people carry on working or go back to work after they retire, but with the low levels of pension savings that we saw in chapter 3 it is likely that many more people in future will have to work for longer out of financial necessity. And people recognise this. The British Social Attitudes Survey carried out annually since 1983 by NatCen, an independent social research agency, shows an increase in the proportion of people who say they expect to retire after 65 for financial reasons, up from 34% in 2008 to 54% in 2011 among those born between 1966 and 1980. There has also been a sharp reduction in the numbers who expect to work after 65 because they enjoy work, from 38% in 2008 to only 8% in 2011.[25]

This is a worry because those who work for financial reasons appear to be less happy. Looking at longitudinal data from ELSA, the survey which asks the same panel of people over 50 about their life, we can see that people who had stayed in work after state pension age due to financial reasons had lower quality of life scores. This was in contrast to those who had made the decision to remain in work for positive reasons, who had higher than average quality of life scores.[26]

Even people in their 80s want to work in order to remain connected and feel valued. I loved the story of 89-year-old Joe Bartley who placed an ad in his local paper seeking part-time work to stop him 'dying from boredom'. He was hired by a local café that recognised their customers often wanted more than a cup of coffee; they wanted a chat, too. Joe had been widowed two years previously and admitted he was lonely, and that the money would also be helpful to pay the rent.[27]

A recent review of research about the views of older workers that looked at a range of studies, including attitude surveys and occupational surveys, found that in general, older workers value many of the same things that younger workers do, such as intellectual stimulation and the chance to work in a sociable environment. Older workers particularly value the social contact they get through work with clients, customers and colleagues.[28] They want the opportunity to use their skills in meaningful ways and engage in work that has meaning to them.

Businesses need these workers, otherwise they risk facing a skills and labour shortage, and for individuals it is both a financial necessity and something they value. So what needs to be done by employers and government to enable more people to remain in work longer?

CREATING AGE FRIENDLY EMPLOYERS

Many companies I have spoken to admit their workforce strategy is focused on how to attract young people into the business. If they have any strategy at all for older workers, it is how to get them to retire! Few have strategies to ensure they retain and recruit older talent. Increasingly, businesses will need to look at how to retain their older workers, recruit older workers and support people later in their careers to train or retrain for new roles and second or third careers. Yet research shows that nearly a quarter (22%) of employers think that their organisation is unprepared for the ageing workforce.[29]

Andy Briggs, the Government's Business Champion for Older Workers and former Chief Executive of UK Insurance at Aviva, believes passionately that, 'Inclusive and diverse businesses are better businesses – they make better decisions and they better represent their customers. If business don't embrace older workers, they will not have the skills and labour they need.' While some businesses are struggling to get the skills and capabilities they need, especially in small- and medium-sized enterprises, not as many companies as he would like to see are embracing older workers as part of the solution.

So how will the world of work need to change to support more people to sustain longer working lives? There are five key ways they can do this (see box below) They need to offer flexibility, hire age-positively, support workers with health conditions and caring responsibilities, support development at all ages and create an age-positive culture.

---

5 ACTIONS TO BE AN AGE-FRIENDLY EMPLOYER

1. Be flexible about flexible working: Offer more kinds of flexibility, manage it well and help people know their options.
2. Hire age positively: Actively target candidates of all ages, and minimise age bias in recruitment processes.
3. Ensure everyone has the health support they need: Offer early and open conversations, and early and sustained access to support for workers with health conditions.
4. Encourage career development at all ages: Provide opportunities for people to develop their careers and plan for the future at mid-life and beyond.
5. Create an age-positive culture: Equip HR professionals and managers to promote an age-positive culture and support interaction across all ages.

Source: Centre for Ageing Better, (2018), Becoming an age-friendly employer.

FLEXIBILITY

Flexible working is important for workers of all ages. However, older workers value it more highly than the general working population[30] and yet the Timewise Flexible Jobs Index 2018 found only 11% of over 6 million job vacancies were advertised as suitable for flexible working, with sector variations ranging from 4% in facilities and construction to 27% in medical and health services.[31]

Being flexible means flexibility around when you work (hours, schedule, breaks), where you work (home, office), what you do (redesigning roles), and how you are expected to work (workplace practices, for instance whether you can take personal calls during work hours). Such flexibilities can help older workers balance caring responsibilities or personal health circumstances and enable a phased transition to retirement.

A number of employee surveys have shown that employees are more likely to stay with employers who offer good quality, flexible working arrangements. However, older workers are not always able to benefit from flexible working. They may lack knowledge about their flexible working options, may assume the right to request flexible working relates only to parents and carers and may not know how to start a discussion in the workplace about changing their work patterns. Employers may share some of these misconceptions and managers may also be resistant to change. Research suggests that many older workers, particularly those in the private sector, don't feel that flexible working options are available or accessible to them.[32]

If older workers are going to remain in work for longer, then more jobs need to be advertised as flexible from the start date, employees of all ages need to be made aware of the right to request flexibility, and line managers need to encourage conversations about the sort of flexibility that might help the person to remain in work and productive. Currently someone must have worked for an employer for at least 26 weeks before being eligible to the right to request flexible working. The government should amend this so there is a right to request flexibility from day 1. If you have caring responsibilities that require flexibility, you simply can't take a job unless you know you can have the flexibility from the start.

HIRE AGE-POSITIVELY

Too many older applicants are frozen out of the job market due to inadequate processes, age bias and a lack of engagement from employers and recruiters. This ultimately disadvantages employers who fail to draw on the experience and abilities of a significant talent pool. In a survey of adults over the age of 50 in

2018 by YouGov for the Centre for Ageing Better, 57% of people who have looked but not applied for a new job since turning 50 felt they would be at a disadvantage in applying for a job because of their age.[33] David's story (see box below) illustrates the challenges faced by those with experience and qualifications in applying for work.

DAVID'S STORY

David is 54 years old and has been out of work for 18 months after being made redundant from his job. He previously taught for 20 years at a local school. In his spare time David puts his skills to good use volunteering for a local history society, while continuing to look for work. David has struggled and failed to gain employment since his redundancy, despite applying for numerous and a wide variety of jobs, registering with lots of recruitment agencies and gaining a number of interviews.

David reports experiencing discrimination in the recruitment process – he feels he was not put forward for certain opportunities as a direct result of his age – but believes that this is under-reported because there is no benefit in complaining. Due to a lack of employment opportunities, David often has to apply for lower level positions and he feels that both his age and professional experience count against him, as he is often perceived with suspicion and as lacking ambition.

Through the Job Centre David enrolled on a self-employment training course run by a local social enterprise. As a result of this course, he was able to pursue a number of opportunities, which unfortunately did not come to fruition. Over the last year, David has been able to gain a few temporary roles, but is increasingly caring for his elderly parents and, while he is still looking for work, David is concentrating on looking after his parents and doing voluntary work, which he can fit around his caring responsibilities.

Elaine Unegbu, Chair of the Greater Manchester Older People's Network, reflected on the attitudes of some employers: 'Somehow there is a blinker as soon as you get to the age of 50 that you cannot retain knowledge ... and employers are losing a lot of people with wisdom, people who have got practical skills, practical knowledge, and that is being lost.'

In the YouGov poll mentioned on page 96, over a quarter (27%) of respondents had been put off jobs since turning 50 as they sounded like they're aimed at younger candidates and nearly one in five (17%) had, or had considered, hiding their age in applying for a job since turning 50. Almost a third (32%) believed they had been turned down for a job because of their age.

Ageism is prevalent in workplaces and appears to combine with other forms of discrimination, such as gender and race, to further disadvantage older women and older women from BAME communities. Under the Equality Act 2010 it is important that age bias, along with these other protected characteristics, is monitored by employers. It is shocking that people are being turned away from jobs because of their age. Experimental studies using fictitious applications have shown that older applicants are less likely to get an interview than younger applicants. In one study the researchers sent nearly 900 matched applications for a variety of low-skilled jobs in the private sector, one set from a 28-year-old White British male and the other from a 50-year-old White British male. The older applicant was over a fifth less likely to be invited for interview compared to the younger applicant. The study also conducted a similar experiment with Black British applicants. They found that the older Black British applicants had a 9 percentage points lower chance of being invited to interview than the older White British applicant. It suggests that when age is combined with ethnicity the level of discrimination faced multiplies.[34]

I find it appalling that some older women I have spoken to have felt the need to make themselves 'look younger' when applying for jobs by changing how they dress or dyeing their hair. The BBC got itself into trouble when it took older women presenters off some of its main programmes. The first such victim was Moira Stuart who, back in 2007, was moved from her Sunday morning news slot. Since then there have been several high-profile cases of older women being replaced on screen. In 2009 Alesha Dixon replaced Arlene Phillips on *Strictly Come Dancing* and, that same year, Miriam O'Reilly and several other women in their 50s were dropped from *Countryfile*. They later successfully sued the BBC for age discrimination. Despite growing criticism of its attitude towards older women, women still only comprise 37% of all on-screen BBC presenters over 50.[35]

The wording and imagery used in advertisements and job descriptions is fundamental in influencing who applies for a role. The Recruitment & Employment Confederation (REC), a network of more than 3500 recruiters, stresses the importance of reflecting on the terminology employers use in job advertisements and job descriptions and asking if it might put certain groups of candidates off. For example, seeking 'a bubbly or effervescent personality', 'lots of energy' or 'a fresh approach and new ways of thinking' may have inadvertent effects upon recruitment by implicitly signalling youth, even though the terms are not directly age-related.[36]

Research has found that attributes stereotypically associated with younger candidates (e.g. being open to new ideas, learning new skills and rapid decision-making) are also viewed more positively in the hiring process than those stereotypically associated with older candidates (e.g. dealing with people politely, settling arguments or carefulness). These 'older' attributes are associated with lower status job roles and recruiters are less likely to select them.[37] There is also a perception that older workers are less productive and less reliable. In another larger study, researchers found that older workers are more consistent, more stable and more highly motivated than younger workers. The study measured the ability of different age cohorts to perform 12 different tasks over 100 days and surmised that the older age cohort had developed strategies over time that helped them solve problems. In other words, they had established coping strategies.[38]

If older workers are to face a fair chance of being hired, recruitment processes need to be monitored for age bias, and active steps taken to ensure that the language and imagery in job adverts is age-neutral, and to eliminate bias at both shortlisting and interview stages. The latter is more difficult as this comes down to some of the biases and stereotypes that recruiters and line managers may have or not be aware that they have. Challenging ageism and creating more positive age-related stereotypes will require a shift in attitudes among recruiters and line managers. Currently there is little likelihood of action being taken against employers that are discriminating on the basis of age, as few cases have been brought by the Equalities and Human Rights Commission and employment tribunals are usually concerned with people who have been dismissed from their job.

SUPPORT WORKERS WITH HEALTH CONDITIONS AND CARING RESPONSIBILITIES

Older workers are more likely to have caring responsibilities or health conditions. Some employers, such as Centrica, are voluntarily taking action to support working age carers and, rather than seeing this as a problem to be avoided, they have introduced a range of policies and support for working carers (see box on page 100). Employers need to start by understanding how many carers they have and what support they might benefit from. They then need to carry out training for line managers and offer networks for working carers, as well as providing or signposting them to information on how to manage the impact of caring on their own finances. In a survey of companies with support for working carers, more than 90% of companies agreed that the policies had improved morale and staff retention. They claimed that this had actually reduced absenteeism and that they got more from these workers.[39]

While it is positive that some employers are taking action to support carers, there needs to be stronger employment rights for carers in the same way that maternity and parental rights have been strengthened and made a huge difference to women's participation in the labour market. Policies are needed to enable working carers to stay in employment for longer and to return to work after a break. This means carers should have the right to some paid leave, as well as longer periods of unpaid leave, with the right to return after a break.

HOW CENTRICA SUPPORTS WORKING CARERS

Centrica was one of the first Employers for Carers, a scheme run by Carers UK for employers who sign up to take action to support carers in the workplace. Over a thousand employees (1 in 36 of its workforce) have now joined its carers' support network. Rights for carers include up to a month's paid care leave, flexibility and carer-inclusive training for line managers. Centrica estimates that it has saved £4.5 million per annum on unplanned absenteeism and £2 million through staff retention since it committed to becoming an Employer for Carers.[40]

A survey of over a thousand people showed one quarter of those aged 55 and over with a health condition who are still in work are considering leaving because of their health. The research also found that workers often put off speaking to employers until the last moment due to poor workplace culture and overly bureaucratic procedures.[41] One person interviewed as part of research to inform Early Help Working Well, Greater Manchester's programme to support those with health conditions to remain in work, said, 'I was only offered a phased return over six weeks and they wouldn't entertain the idea of letting me come back part-time due to my health. I couldn't even walk the distance between the car park and my office at that point. It was impossible.'

Due to the long-term and slow onset of some health conditions, older workers may not identify they have a disability and may therefore miss out on some of the legal protections and support available to employees with disabilities. Older workers are also often afraid to raise issues about health conditions and need to feel supported if they do disclose health conditions. A workplace culture in which health and wellbeing issues are openly discussed and supported can also help people with health conditions to ask for the help and support they need, without fear of reprisal, judgement or job loss. Early access to support, small adjustments to the workplace and working patterns, and empathetic management are crucial to enabling people to manage their health at work and remain in employment.

Many of the adjustments that people need are small and inexpensive. If not covered under the employer's obligation to provide reasonable adjustments, employees can apply for an Access to Work grant to fund practical support in the workplace. This government-funded grant can then be paid to the person with additional needs (to cover the costs of adapting a vehicle needed to get to work, for example) or to the employer directly (such as purchasing specialist equipment or software for the workplace). Greater awareness and promotion of this grant is needed.

Technology could also assist so more of us might be able to do jobs that we didn't think possible at older ages. Exoskeleton suits might conjure up images of the Bionic Man, but they are becoming more prevalent and can enable physically demanding roles to be done more easily and with less damage to our health, helping people with health conditions or disabilities to carry out jobs they would currently have to give up. Projects like the Aura Power suit – an exoskeleton suit which enhances human strength – could help people in manual and physical jobs carry on working without getting musculoskeletal problems from heavy lifting. The Haneda Airport in Tokyo has used similar technology to enable older workers to move heavier luggage and reduce the risk of injury, for example. On the other hand, deployed too quickly, such suits could result in people losing muscle strength.

Companies that harness technology and use it to change the work environment to enable older workers to continue to be productive are likely to see the rewards. Upon realising that its workforce's average age was approaching 47, car manufacturer

THE AGE OF AGEING BETTER?

BMW made small, cost-effective changes to the work environment in its Bavarian factory, resulting in greater productivity, decreased sickness leave and improved worker morale. Although it made over 70 small changes to the factory's design and environment, this cost less than 40,000 euros and increased the productivity of all staff by 7% in a year.[42] Employers that support employees with caring responsibilities and health conditions to remain in work will be rewarded with a productivity dividend.

Workplace initiatives like Time to Change (a campaign to de-stigmatise mental health) and Mental Health First Aid (a programme to train staff as first responders for colleagues with mental health issues), as well as a greater focus on wellbeing at work, are likely to help reduce the impact of stress and enable those with mental health issues to get support to remain in work. For those who are later in their working lives, burnout from continuous stress in frontline roles like teaching, social work and nursing might also need to be addressed to prevent people leaving work involuntarily, particularly as early retirement options are no longer widely available. An evaluation of pre-retirement courses which provide psychological and emotional support found that people re-evaluated their work-life balance, which led to reductions in job involvement for those with high levels before the course. Very high levels of job involvement have been shown to lead to burnout.[43] Alternatively, earlier career conversations could identify other (less stressful) roles and provide people with retraining options to pursue other career opportunities.

SUPPORT DEVELOPMENT AT ALL AGES

The prospect that more of us will live to 100 will also mean more of us restarting second or third careers later in life. The notion of positions being graduate-level entry or 'junior' positions being for school leavers needs to change. Internships, apprenticeships and entry-level roles to a career need to be equally available to someone starting out again at 50 with another 20 years of work ahead of them as a 20-year-old who is unlikely to stay in the same career for the next 50 or more years. Training is vital to this, and yet older workers are less likely to get the same opportunities for training and development as their younger counterparts. The UK has the third-worst rate of job-related training in the OECD for over 50s.[44] Often the focus is on teaching technical skills, but these become obsolete very quickly, and need to be learnt and relearnt, often on the job. The skills that are important to maintaining resilience and sustaining a longer working life may be softer skills such as adaptability and flexibility.

The 100-year life also presents a challenge to the current patterns of progression and promotion.[45] The traditional link between age, seniority and pay may be broken with people starting out again in mid-life. The expectation of career paths needs to change, with greater opportunities for retraining and progression throughout the life course. If young people starting out in work today are to sustain much longer working lives, employers and government will need to: increase investment in retraining and reskilling people; create more opportunities for life-long learning, on the job training and development opportunities; and redesign apprenticeships and internships to suit those who are changing careers in mid-life or later in life.

There is currently very low uptake of apprenticeships amongst the over 50s and yet there is a huge underspend on the Apprenticeship Levy (a compulsory charge made on large employers), in part because of the limits on how the funding can be spent, including that the money has to be spent within two years. This could be remodelled to give greater flexibility both to how the funding is spent and to create an apprenticeship-like model that is more suited to older workers looking to retrain or start over. This could mean reforming the Apprenticeship Levy so that the funding is not only spent on entry-level workplace training schemes as now, but also on other training schemes which might be more attractive and relevant to those who are retraining later in life. A new government scheme announced in 2018 with £100 million of funding called the National Retraining Scheme is designed to provide (mainly) online training support to people who are at risk of redundancy because of the rapid technological changes in the economy. It will need to be carefully designed if it is to engage older workers who may not have digital skills or may not recognise their need to retrain.

The 100-year life will also require people to rethink their work-life balance across the life course in order to preserve health and vitality to sustain a longer working life. Some companies are offering career 'learning breaks' or reintroducing sabbaticals, giving people time out to think through the next stage of their career, or to retrain or refresh their skills. Older workers can also play an important role as mentors, either for younger apprentices or by passing on their knowledge and skills to future generations. But it doesn't need to be one-way. Younger people have skills and knowledge that they can share with older colleagues in return.

Some forward-thinking companies, which have recognised that the retirement of highly skilled and experienced professionals poses a risk to their business, are looking to find ways of not only retaining these staff, but also offering them roles as mentors and trainers to ensure their skills and knowledge are passed on to the next generation of workers. I spoke recently to BAE Systems who face a challenge with a high proportion of their highly trained engineers approaching retirement. The company offers a generous pension, so there is little incentive to stay working longer, but it is beginning to think about how it might engage these individuals, to explore ways they could stay on, potentially in other roles or on flexible contracts. These roles also help the individual to make the transition to retirement in a gradual way, avoiding the cliff edge. They feel their knowledge and experience is valued and they can leave in a planned way where the work they have contributed is handed over.

Some organisations such as Legal and General (see box on page 105) have also introduced the idea of a mid-life MOT, which I discussed in chapter 3, for their workers. They see this as a way of supporting and valuing workers in mid-life, and being able to have conversations about their careers, and options to retrain and change roles.

LEGAL AND GENERAL MID-LIFE MOT

Legal and General, a large financial services company, ran a midlife MOT pilot in 2017. They invited staff between the ages of 45 and 55 to take part, and more than 50 employees participated. They ran four workshops in two of their offices. Debt, saving and financial management were covered in their financial wellness seminar. Another session on pensions tested out a new tool to help people visualise the retirement they wanted and see how much more they would need to save to achieve that income. As well as highlighting the importance of financial preparation in later life, other workshops concentrated on health and wellbeing (with employees being given access to a one-to-one biometric assessment and an app to encourage regular reviews of their health and wellbeing) and a work-life assessment (to find out more about how the workplace is changing and what options are open to people).

The pilots were informed by feedback from participants and, according to a post-workshop review conducted two months later, more than 90% of employees found the workshops useful, and most found the health and wellbeing workshop informative. Nearly 90% felt informed about their current pension value, but just 60% felt they knew how much money they would need in retirement.[46]

AN AGE-POSITIVE CULTURE

Older workers want to work in organisations which demonstrate openness and foster intergenerational working. A study of employer and employee views by the Chartered Institute of Personnel and Development, the professional body for HR professionals, found that some older workers feel that their managers are not doing enough to make mixed-age teams work successfully.[47] This often comes down to the ability of line managers to effectively manage age-diverse teams and to relate to staff who may be older than them. And yet if the diverse views and perspectives of people of different ages and stages can be harnessed by creating a positive age culture that values everyone, then this can have benefits for the productivity, creativity and performance of teams.

Diversity and inclusion policies and training, especially common in large organisations, need to include age as a protected characteristic. Employers also need to change managers' attitudes and beliefs about older workers. Although there are examples of employers providing age-diversity awareness training, there is a complete lack of research on how effective it is. Some businesses have created age champions who are visible leaders and who raise awareness of age-diversity issues. Other companies have networks or forums for older workers to meet and share concerns, and to make suggestions to the management of the organisation about changes or improvements that would make them more engaged.

Employers need to ensure older workers are not overlooked for development opportunities or progression, or systematically discriminated against in performance reviews. This will require employers to collect and monitor data by age. Most companies do not monitor age in the same way they do other diversity characteristics, such as gender and race. Transparency and monitoring data are important first steps in identifying whether processes and pay are fair, and opportunities for progression equally available. Making this a requirement might bring this issue into the light and shame those companies that are not doing enough. Look at the shift that is taking place on the gender pay gap since the government required all employers with more than 250 employees to publish this data.

Within the Civil Service there is a highly standardised performance rating system and yet despite this the Department for Work and Pensions (which publishes its data) found that older workers are systematically underrepresented in the highest performance markings. A quarter of those aged 25 to 34 were said to have exceeded their performance goals at review, compared to just 14% of those aged 55 to 64. While more than a quarter of staff are over 55, less than 10% of promotions go to this age group.[48] It is possible that older workers are not performing as well as younger workers, but other research suggests that older workers perform as well as younger workers at a range of tasks, welcome the opportunity to learn new skills, are often better at negotiation and resolving inter-personal problems, and report higher engagement and loyalty to their employer.[49] Such a systematic difference could also reflect the attitudes of line managers or suggest that the skills and experience of older workers are not being measured or are undervalued. Analysis of business data in the US by Mercer, a global professional services firm, indicates individual performance measures fail to account for the indirect contribution that older workers make to team performance, for example, through coaching and knowledge transfer or the stability more typical of groups with older workers.[50]

Far from the growth in older workers being a threat to the jobs of younger workers, there is a real and pending risk that as the 1960s baby boomers leave the workforce, the UK will face a labour and skills shortage. It will need employers to radically shift their focus and practices to create more age-friendly employment opportunities by: embracing flexibility in all its forms; eliminating age bias in the recruitment process; supporting workers with health conditions and caring responsibilities to manage these and remain in work; investing in the training and progression of older workers; and creating an age-positive culture in which the diverse contributions of workers of all ages are harnessed.

Does there remain a risk that more older workers will be a drag on productivity? The research I have touched on above suggests, at least at team level, performance can be enhanced by having age diversity, but let's look in more detail at the productivity challenge of an ageing workforce.

THE PRODUCTIVITY CHALLENGE OF AN AGEING WORKFORCE

The Conservative government published its Industrial Strategy in 2017.[51] It stated that, 'Without action, an ageing population could reduce the size of our workforce and lead to lower productivity.' The UK in particular has a productivity challenge compared to other industrialised countries, with outputs and profit per worker remaining stagnant. A review of the evidence by the Department of Business, Energy and Industrial Strategy suggested that firm-level management and leadership capability, as well as the adoption and diffusion of technology, were most important in explaining productivity differences between businesses which were technically similar in terms of size or industry.[52] The number of older workers did not appear to be a factor at the level of individual firms.

The productivity challenge for the national economy is the gap in economic activity between those aged 50 to state pension age and younger age groups, which is not fully shown in the data. The Annual Population Survey shows us that between July 2018 and June 2019, there were 12.6 million people aged 50–64 in the UK. Of these, about 9.4 million were economically active. More than 7 million were employees, a further 1.7 million were self-employed and 266,000 were looking for work. However, there are nearly 3.3 million who were 'economically inactive'.[53] By the time they're 64, more than 60% of people are economically inactive.[54] A 1% increase in the number of people in work aged 50–64 could increase GDP by around £5.7 billion per year and have a positive impact on income tax and National Insurance contributions of around £800 million per year.[55] Currently, this rapid drop-off in the proportion of people in work starts from the age of 55 onwards (see the chart on page 109), with 79% of men employed at the age of 55, but only 68% at the age of 60.

For women this difference is even starker, with 73% employed at the age of 55, and 57% at 60.[56] These people are not earning and are therefore paying less in income tax and National Insurance. They may also be spending less, reducing the amount going into the local economy and collected in VAT. It is this gap that worries the economists and the Government.

The Government's Industrial Strategy went on to set out its vision for the future: 'British businesses will have redesigned jobs and workplaces to better use their older workers' experience, enabling individuals to keep active and stay in work. Workers will have more flexibility to help balance their work with caring responsibilities. Younger generations will be able to plan for their longer careers with confidence.' The expectation is that if more people are working, this increases the amount of tax revenues, generates economic growth through higher consumer spending and reduces the amount spent on benefits. Higher employment rates of skilled and experienced workers can also contribute to economic growth and higher productivity.

So, as well as benefits to the individual, financially, socially and psychologically, more people working longer generates economic and financial benefits for all of us.

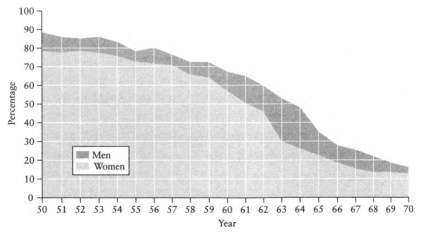

Employment rate by single year of age and sex.
Source: Annual Population Survey, June 2015–July 2016.

WHO MAKES UP THIS 'GAP' AND WHAT NEEDS TO CHANGE TO CLOSE IT?

In 2018–19, there were 3.5 million people out of work, with only 8% saying they were actively seeking work[57] – which usually means they are on Jobseeker's Allowance or Universal Credit, the controversial new single monthly payment that replaces six previous benefits if you are out of work or on a low income and is being rolled out across the UK. Those who are out of work and claiming benefits at older ages are usually on Employment and Support Allowance, an incapacity benefit which requires people to undertake a work capability assessment to judge their ability to work. Employment and Support Allowance has a higher financial entitlement and fewer conditions than Jobseeker's Allowance, so someone with a disability over the age of 50 is unlikely to claim Jobseeker's Allowance or Universal Credit if they can claim Employment and Support Allowance. As we will see in chapter 6, there are high levels of early disability, particularly among lower socio-economic groups. Disability-free life expectancy is lowest in the most deprived areas, but there are only 16 local areas (out of more than 200) in England in which both males and females at birth have a disability-free life expectancy of more than 65. This means that in most places a majority of people already have a disability before they are 65, so they are often able to claim some form of incapacity benefit without a requirement to be looking for work.[58] Although theoretically the benefits system is supposed to be the same at all ages, few economically inactive people aged 50-64 are on Jobseeker's Allowance, which would require them to 'sign on' and attend work-related programmes.

Even though the numbers actively seeking work are low, around 1 million people in this age range are estimated to be 'involuntarily workless' – that is they *want to work* but are out of work for a range of reasons, including ill health or disability, caring responsibilities and redundancy.[59] I've already briefly looked at what employers can do to support people with health conditions and caring responsibilities remain in work, so let's turn to those who are out of work, and what is needed to help them return to work and to close the economic activity gap.

FALLING OUT OF WORK AT OLDER AGES

Health conditions are one of the leading reasons people leave the labour market before state pension age. The two leading health conditions for stopping work at any age are mental health and musculoskeletal conditions (known as MSK). The majority of people aged between 50 and state pension age who are not in work due to a disability say it is due to musculoskeletal problems.[60] Many of these problems are due to the impact of work itself.

Heavy manual work takes a toll on people's physical health and can mean they experience disability earlier, impacting their ability to continue in work. The decline in industries such as mining and manufacturing in the UK has reduced the number of people working in 'dangerous' jobs. Improvements in compliance with environmental standards and health and safety at work regulations over the past three decades have also reduced problems, with a halving of fatal accidents at work between 1981 and 2016[61], and a 44% reduction in workplace accidents between 2000 and 2017.[62] But office-based jobs have a negative impact on health, too. Sedentary work, along with the car, is one of the major contributing factors to obesity, lack of fitness and back pain.

However, people often have multiple conditions and it seems that MSK is the condition they cite as the reason for stopping work, although they may have other related or contributing conditions. There is also some evidence of the co-occurrence of mental and physical health issues. According to the Health and Safety Executive, nearly 600,000 workers in Great Britain suffered from work related stress, depression or anxiety in 2017-2018 and 15.4 million working days were lost due to this. Workers in the education sector were the most likely to be off work with mental health problems.[63]

Disability and illness that limits people's ability to work affects people in lower-income jobs disproportionately. Recent analysis by Les Mayhew, Professor of Statistics at City, University of London, found that back-to-work policies for people over 50 are less likely to be effective given the prevalence of disability and the link with economic inactivity. More important for improving economic activity rates for lower income groups is preventing early-onset disability. Some research has also suggested that the deprivation of the area has a greater influence on disability rates than job type, with some manual workers in affluent areas having a similar or higher disability-free life expectancy as someone in a managerial or professional role in a more deprived area.[64] The proportion of people out of work due to ill-health is higher among those in the lowest wealth bracket compared to those in the highest wealth bracket. Among men aged 55-59 with a health condition, 30% in the poorest fifth of the population are not working, compared to 3% in the richest group. The difference is even more pronounced for women: among women aged 55-59 with a health problem in the poorest fifth, 42% are not in work, compared to just 4% of women with a health problem in the richest group.[65]

In addressing these barriers to work it is important to recognise their complexity and that fixing them will often require a joined-up approach between health and employment services. The NHS Long Term Plan published in 2019 set out a five-year plan for how the NHS is going to change in order to meet the current health needs of the population in England.[66] Recognising the importance of rapid access to physiotherapy to enable people with MSK problems to return quickly to work, the NHS proposes to introduce first-contact appointments with a physio in general practice for those with MSK conditions to speed up the process.

We know from research that it is less likely for older workers who are made redundant, for whatever reason, including on health grounds, to work again. More than 40% of people over 50 who are unemployed have been so for over 12 months, nearly double the percentage of 25 to 49-year-olds who have been out of work for more than a year.[67] There is some evidence from the Department for Work and Pensions that about a quarter of those

THE WORLD OF WORK

who are between 50 and state pension age and unemployed were made redundant from their last job.[68] How does employment support need to change to enable more of these people to return to work?

EMPLOYMENT SUPPORT

Whatever the cause of people being economically inactive, it is critical that employment support is effective in supporting people to return to work, yet older jobseekers have more difficulty than any other group in returning to work. Analysis of the government's Work Programme, which is a programme of commissioned support helping the long-term unemployed return to work, shows just 21% of people over the age of 50 who were long-term unemployed ended up in a long-term job – a success rate of just over one in five.[69] This is despite the fact that the providers get paid more for getting people into work and keeping them there. Those over 60 with a mental health problem are the least likely to return to work after the government's Work Programme, which is lower than for other age groups with mental health problems and for others of the same age but with different health problems or disabilities.[70]

The barriers to returning to employment for this group are many and various. Insight work by the Centre for Ageing Better with people in their 50s who were out of work in neighbourhoods across Greater Manchester identified multiple problems. Nearly everyone we spoke to was dealing with a health condition (physical or mental) and often providing care and support to a relative as well. Many were struggling to find a job, or at least a job description, that they could apply their skills and experience to in the modern-day labour market, and too few jobs offered any flexibility. Support around employment and skills was frequently felt to be unsuitable for someone of 'their age'. As a result of these significant challenges, and often many failed attempts to return to work, many had written themselves off as too old to work. Stephen, who we met in Brinnington,

113

Stockport, considered himself retired – at the age of 47. A lack of local economic opportunities and other environmental factors, such as lack of transport links or the costs of public transport, also presented a challenge.[71]

Many of you will be familiar with the story depicted in the film *I Daniel Blake*. It tells the story of Daniel, a 59-year-old carpenter from Newcastle, who suffers a heart attack. Following a work capability assessment, he is not deemed eligible for Employment and Support Allowance. The film documents his fight with the bureaucratic benefits system and the challenges of living with no income or pension. The issues in the film are reflected in the stories of real people who struggle to navigate the benefits and employment support system. I recently received a letter from Jenny, a former teacher and librarian, whose story (see box below) illustrates the challenges of worklessness and the problems with employment support.

JENNY'S STORY

Jenny (name changed) cared for her father full-time for two years and after his death was reliant on Jobseeker's Allowance. At 60 years old she tried hard to get work. While potential employers were impressed with her qualifications, she lacked recent work experience and was struggling with some of the job applications, which were online. She won't get her state pension until she is 66 and has only small occupational pensions from when she was working, lives in social housing and is reliant on Housing Benefit. The work coach at the Job Centre made her do a four-week, low-paid physically demanding job for the Royal Mail. The council was not informed in time that this was only a casual job and started charging her full rent. Her Housing Benefit stopped, and she wasn't eligible for Working Tax Credit. As a result, she got into rent arrears and debt. She also recounts how, on another occasion, she was given 48 hours' notice to attend a competitive recruitment process involving role plays and snap interviews on what, even the

---

recruiters conceded, would be a long day. She was exhausted and refused to attend, and as a result was sanctioned for three months. She has now successfully applied for Employment and Support Allowance with the help of her GP.

She wrote powerfully: 'All this is having a detrimental effect on my mental and physical wellbeing; the relentless attrition over where the next penny is coming from, the panic attacks if I should lose money or even a bus ticket that I know I can't replace, the neglect of my health, the risks to my home, being forcibly marginalised from society … Is it any wonder when you're daily reminded that society has no use for you, that you are a burden on the state and are likely to become even worse as you get older and less able? I feel that my life expectancy is being compromised, that continual anxiety is damaging the quality of my life, if it can be viewed as a life rather than a precarious existence. But the worst part of all of this is knowing that being on the Employment and Support Allowance is only a brief respite and that the fundamental problem still remains – I am out of work, over 60 and no-one wants to hire me.'

According to Jenny the current system 'punishes the old in its inflexibility of procedure, unrealistic expectations and the sanctions.' Her experience of Job Centres and the benefits system is a very powerful example of how the current system of employment support is failing people who are out of work, particularly those in later life, who find it harder than any other age group to return to work.

There is a need for new models of employment support that are tailored to the over 50s, which are more personalised and holistic, and which recognise the multiple issues that people at this age face when trying to get work. This may require, for example, job coaches to be trained to specialise in support for over 50s and employment support services to be integrated better with health services. Ideally the approach should also be local, so that those working in Job Centres can build up relationships with employers who are willing to take on these older job seekers and identify opportunities in the local labour market. The government also needs to consider whether to provide stronger incentives to employers to take on these workers. As we considered in the chapter on money, there may also need to be increased flexibility in the benefits system to enable people to take on part-time roles or limit the roles they take to those that are 'appropriate' given their health and caring responsibilities. For example, jobs might be restricted to locations that are within easy travel distance or offer particular hours of work (i.e. not shift work).

Closing the employment gap for older workers is vital to boost productivity. Older job seekers often face multiple barriers and a new approach to employment support for people at this age and stage of life is needed, particularly as changes in the labour market might mean more older workers being made redundant in future.

CHANGES IN THE LABOUR MARKET

Large lay-offs in the 1980s and 1990s in heavy industries such as mining and manufacturing, due to companies moving overseas, resulted in people (largely men) being made redundant. Many of those in their 50s and 60s at the time never returned to work and many were able to claim incapacity benefits as they had poor health or disabilities which affected their ability to work. Technology and automation are predicted to result in large numbers of existing workers being made redundant. There is lots of speculation about how artificial intelligence (AI) and robotics will replace human workers in the future. These developments are not some sci-fi future. For some medical conditions it is already possible for computers using AI to diagnose patients more accurately and more quickly than doctors and health care professionals. The work of legal assistants and paralegals is already being replaced by computers, which can search and review large volumes of documentation more efficiently. While we are already seeing how automatic self-checkouts are reducing the numbers of retail staff in stores (the majority of whom were traditionally older women), these are being replaced by jobs in warehouses and vans, due to the growth in online shopping and home delivery. There is a risk that the next wave of technology – driverless vans and drones – will replace these jobs in turn.

When I spoke to Matthew Taylor, Chief Executive of the Royal Society for the Encouragement of Arts, Manufactures and Commerce (RSA), who led a government review on self-employment, the gig economy and the future of work, he suggested that the hollowing out effect will mainly affect mid-level jobs. By this he meant that technology with allow less skilled people to do the things that previously only higher skilled workers could do. Because older workers are concentrated at the top and bottom end of the labour market, they are less likely to be adversely affected by this. In terms of the timeframe, he suggested these technological changes will impact on the opportunities for future cohorts in the next decade or more and it will be important that they are supported to return to work following redundancy.

What support is currently available and how effective is it? Job Centre Plus provides a rapid response service in some instances of large-scale redundancies, but this is generic and the service isn't necessarily able to respond to the diverse needs of the workforce. Large corporations will sometimes purchase a private outplacement provision for anyone they are making redundant, but access to this and its quality varies hugely. It is vital that those who are being made redundant from jobs that are being replaced by technology or are no longer required due to innovation in the market, are supported to access new work opportunities. This will mean workers of all ages accessing on-the-job training to keep their knowledge and skills up-to-date or retraining to take on roles in other sectors or companies. For example, changes in the construction industry could result in many fewer physical jobs on building sites as more modular homes are built in high-precision factories. These jobs will require a very different skill set. There is a need to develop and test new approaches to redeployment, including for those being made redundant from small- and medium-enterprises in the supply chain of large companies which are closing down.

These ideas are not going to work, though, if there are no jobs to be had in the local labour market. Alongside these changes there needs to be investment in economic development to create alternative job opportunities for those who do not want to or are unable to relocate. There is a risk that in some of these areas, well-paid and secure jobs are replaced with insecure, low-skill and low-pay jobs, so it is critical that we improve the quality of jobs by generating economic growth in sectors that require higher skilled roles.

THE QUALITY OF WORK MATTERS

The quality of work matters. Research indicates that being in poor quality work can be as detrimental to your health as not working.[72] In general, poor-quality work is work that is insecure, low paid, where there is little or no control over your work and a lack of progression and opportunity. For those in low-pay and low-skilled work, the risk is that they never progress and remain stuck in poor quality work for longer, thus there is a negative impact on their health and their financial situation, which puts them at high risk of poor outcomes in later life.

Matthew Taylor, whom I mentioned earlier, looked at the features of 'good work' as part of his review for government. When I spoke with him, he explained that judging the quality of work was subjective and depends on circumstances and preferences. He shared this example: 'A 19-year-old delivery driver probably feels perfectly happy, but if you'd been doing it for five years and couldn't get anything else, you'd feel differently about it.' He went on to describe some basic objective measures, such as pay and conditions, and whether people are treated fairly. Then there are secondary factors, such as whether people feel trusted to make decisions, whether they are listened to as a human being and respected, whether there is a community at work that is sociable and inclusive, and finally, whether there are opportunities for personal growth, development and promotion.

It is imperative that we don't just measure the success of the economy by the number of jobs created or indeed the levels of employment, but that the quality of those jobs is measured. In the final report of Taylor's review, he recommended that there needs to be better quality metrics for good work, which the government committed to developing. The RSA and Carnegie Trust proposed seven measures of job quality, covering: terms of employment (e.g. minimum hours); pay and benefits; health, safety and psychosocial wellbeing; job design and nature of work; social support and cohesion; voice and representation; and work-life balance.[73] However, it does seem that the youngest and oldest age groups are least likely to be in good quality work. In an analysis of the 2012 Skills and Employment Survey, which defined a good quality job as one which utilises your strengths, involves you in decision-making and has performance-related pay, it was those in their 30s who were most likely to be in good quality work.[74]

There is a view that changes in the nature of work are disproportionately affecting millennials, and that while older workers enjoy the security of permanent employment status, younger workers are left to take poorly paid and insecure work with no prospects of progression. So what is the reality?

There are a number of different types of insecure or flexible work. Zero-hour contracts mean there is no guarantee of a minimum number of hours that someone will work in a particular week or month. This means that the employer can match capacity to demand, for example, if they have some busy shifts one week, they can get extra workers to work for those hours. These workers are definitely employed and therefore do have employment rights. However, for the individual it can mean income can fluctuate from week to week, making budgeting impossible.

The gig economy is a term used to describe work that originally was literally a 'gig', a one-off paid session. It is now used to refer to the growth in all sorts of work provided by freelancers or independent contractors. There is currently an incentive for companies to make people self-employed and so avoid having to pay tax, holiday pay and pension contributions. Controversially, drivers for companies like Uber and Deliveroo are also classed as gig workers. Uber doesn't own the vehicles or 'employ' the drivers. Recent court cases and tribunals have sought to clarify the status of some workers who are currently being classified as self-employed. The implications of these cases and other individual tribunal hearings are still unclear.

The challenge here is not only the unpredictability of the availability of work and therefore income, but also these workers do not have any employment rights or access to pensions. Current estimates suggest that between a quarter and a third of the self-employed are saving into a private pension. At present, auto enrolment does not apply to the self-employed and as a result these workers are more likely to find themselves without a decent income in later life. However, even if gig workers were classified by their employers as workers, most would not meet the earning threshold for auto enrolment. In a 2019 online survey of over 2,000 adults over the age of 18, 45% of both those who were self-employed and non-standard workers, such as those on temporary or zero-hour contracts, said 'they sometimes have trouble meeting basic living costs because their income varies month to month', compared to just 17% of 'typical' employees.[75] Self-employed people were also more concerned about their current income than those classed as 'non-standard' workers (on temporary, or zero-hour contracts). Only one in five (21%) felt their work provided enough money to maintain a decent standard of living, compared to 38% of non-standard workers. While 44% of those who were 'typical' employees or self-employed said they didn't expect to have enough in private pensions and other savings to maintain a decent standard of living in retirement, over half (52%) of 'non-standard' workers thought the same.

Finally, the sharing economy refers to new business models based on charging for things you own that were not previously commodities; for example, Airbnb enables you to rent out spare rooms or schemes like Getaround allow you to rent your car when you're not using it. For those who rely on this sort of work as their main income, these new types of role and employment status have a lot of downsides, but they do offer flexibility and therefore may be positive for those looking for side gigs to allow them to pursue other work, top up a pension or balance other commitments, such as caring. There are examples of where the sharing economy has been embraced by older generations and, for example, more than one in 10 of Airbnb hosts are over aged 60, according to the company.[76] This also reflects some of the patterns of home ownership I look at in the chapter on housing.

Data from the British Social Attitudes Survey suggests that there has been an increase in the proportion of people at older ages who do not feel secure in their jobs compared to those at younger ages.[77] This may simply be because they have previously enjoyed greater job security, rather than that they are more affected by these changes in work. Between 2001 and 2016, there was a 69% increase in so-called 'solo' self-employed (SSE), mostly freelancers. There has also been a more general growth in the numbers of self-employed (including those who have employees). The rise in self-employment is not only impacting on younger workers. A quarter of the solo self-employed are in their 50s[78] and the numbers of self-employed people aged 65 years and older rose from 159,000 to 469,000 between 2001 and 2016.[79] A high proportion of freelancers are professionals: almost half are highly qualified and one in four have a skilled trade – equivalent to 1.1 million people.

As if to highlight the issues at hand, the day I met up with Matthew Taylor, Uber drivers were protesting in central London. We discussed the challenges of making the gig economy work. Taylor defends platform-based work and gig work, such as food delivery or transport, that is initiated or completed through online platforms like Uber or Deliveroo, arguing it often provides two-way flexibility that certain people want for any number of reasons, including older people who may want to work but don't need to maximise their income. But he recognises that it could have a wider 'chilling' effect on regulations in the labour market by watering down the protections that employed workers enjoy.

He believes that most people who work in non-standard contracts want that. He disagrees with some on the Left who argue that those who are happy with zero hours contracts are an example of 'false consciousness': in other words, they don't know they could have better employment rights. Some polling suggests that there are generally high levels of satisfaction among those working in the gig economy, but it depends on how much of a person's income is derived from the gig economy.[80]

Taylor sees reasons to be optimistic. He notes that there are higher levels of employment than ever before and a lot fewer workless households. Most people in work are happy with their work and there hasn't been a very steep rise in zero-hour contracts. On the other hand, living standards have frozen and the cyclical rise in self-employment following a recession has not recovered; something Taylor thinks could be a long-term change in the economy. He recognises that addressing these structural issues in the economy will be challenging, but that ways of improving living standards for workers need to be found. He mentioned examples such as shared ownership models, where the dividends of higher productivity from investments in capital and technology benefit the workers rather than shareholders and income from shares supplements wage income for more people. He suggested it may also require us to consider more radical proposals, such as a shorter working week – but where pay is sufficient to enable people to afford a reasonable standard of living.

The government were consulting on proposals in response to the Taylor Review at the time of writing, considering whether workers should be compensated for shifts cancelled at the last minute, and additional protection for workers who reject shifts, among other proposals.[81] But the pace of change in the job market is outstripping the response and many workers, young and old, risk experiencing forced flexibility, which leaves them in insecure work and low incomes which are not only detrimental to their current health and wealth, but may leave them in an ever more precarious position in later life. If there continues to be a growth in flexible working patterns, this could be a good thing if *it is by choice* and those who opt for these types of working arrangements are not disadvantaged, either in the employment rights they enjoy or their ability to benefit from a pension. However, the reality at the moment is that people get stuck in low-paid and insecure work with few opportunities for progression. This is a huge risk for current and future generations. A life of low-paid work is likely to result in poorer health, earlier exit from the labour market, fewer, if any, savings, and poorer outcomes in later life.

WHAT NEEDS TO CHANGE

Whatever the future holds, one thing is certain: that the workforce will be, on average, older than today's workforce. Not only are we living longer, but we will also need, and in many cases want, to work longer. Much longer working lives will be the reality for many people and this will require changes to the world of work. Some employers have woken up to this new reality and are beginning to notice the change in the age profile of their own workforce as the impact of policies, such as the removal of the default retirement age, increases in the age at which people receive the state pension and the closing of most defined benefit pensions, are impacting people's decisions about when to stop work.

Labour and skills shortages will make retaining older workers a necessity for all employers in the future and there may be competitive advantage in doing so. There are likely to be general labour shortages as each year more workers leave due to retirement than enter from school or university, allaying any concerns that older workers are taking jobs from younger workers, for which there is no basis in evidence anyway. Tighter immigration controls could mean that the gap won't easily be filled by recruiting internationally. Workforce strategies solely focused on recruiting new (young) talent are not likely to provide sufficient skilled workers. Skills shortages mean employers are concerned about losing experience and are starting to consider how to retain and transfer the knowledge and expertise of older workers in critical roles.

Those employers who do recognise the change need to act to get ahead of their competitors. More age diverse teams can have positive benefits if the ideas and different perspectives are harnessed to deliver improvements in performance, productivity and innovation. Some leading employers are making changes to become age-friendly. This requires collaborative and inclusive workplace cultures that value difference and can harness the experience, talent and skills of younger and older workers alike. By making adjustments to the work environment and job roles, employers can help support people with health conditions and caring responsibilities.

These changes may be driven by individuals making different choices and demanding changes from their employers, and employers responding to the changing dynamics of the labour market. But they are more likely to come about, and come about more quickly, if Government takes action. The Government should: require employers to be more transparent about age inequality, as it has done successfully on gender; provide incentives and support to enable employers to address the barriers that those who have health conditions and disabilities face; introduce employment rights for working carers; and require jobs to be flexible from day one, not after a six-week wait.

And yet there will continue to be many people who are simply unable to keep working longer due to health conditions, disability or caring responsibilities. As the type and location of jobs changes in response to global economic forces, political changes, climate change and rapid technological developments, some workers will find it harder to adapt or to return to work following redundancy. It is vital to economic growth that we close the gap in the economic activity between older and younger ages. This will require action to improve employment support for older job seekers.

Technology is either painted as being the answer to all society's problems or the cause of them. Predictions about the impact on the world of work will no doubt be proven wrong in many respects. However, there are opportunities for technology to be harnessed for good. It can enable those currently excluded from work to access employment opportunities by augmenting or assisting with tasks that are physically or cognitively demanding. It can enable flexibility; look, for example, at how improvements in connectivity, cloud technology and video communications have enabled the recent explosion in remote working. Technological developments and automation may also reduce the negative impacts of some types of work on health, thus keeping people healthier and able to work for longer.

But technology, automation and AI are also predicted to put many people out of work. Employers and government must provide effective support for those who are made redundant to retrain and get back to work quickly. This might require stronger incentives for employers to fund support for workers at risk of redundancy to increase the likelihood of them being retrained and redeployed. It will also require increased investment in life-long and work-based training. Personal learning accounts which provide individuals with a budget for training, like they have introduced in Singapore, could be one solution and may be a better way of using the Apprenticeship Levy.

Technology is also a significant factor in the growth of the gig economy, with online networks connecting consumers with service providers or workers. As we have seen, the rise in self-employment and gig work is not only impacting younger workers. Older workers are also shifting to these new types of role. Time will tell what the long-term impact these changes will have on people's health, wellbeing and financial security. For now, to create a level playing field, the priority must be to extend auto enrolment in pensions to the self-employed, as well as clarifying the employment rights of these workers.

Sooner or later most of us will stop paid work for one reason or another and 'retire'. And in order to ensure life doesn't stop when the job does, we need to think carefully about what we do with our time. The next chapter looks at how we are spending this time.

5

What we do with our time

'Ideal condition of old age: physical comfort; independence;
the power to give as well as to receive.'[1]

Charles Booth (1898)

What does the word 'retirement' conjure up for you? A picture
of a wealthy pensioner cruising, boozing, having a good time and
squandering the kids' inheritance? Or a reward for the hard graft
put in during a working life? Perhaps you can't wait to give up
work and have time to do the things you enjoy. Or perhaps the idea
brings on a sense of dread, a fear about withdrawal, boredom or
loss of status. When going through my father-in-law's belongings
after he died, my husband came across a hand-written note with
five definitions of 'retire' none of which are very positive:

1. To give up, or to cause a person to give up his work,
   especially on reaching retirement age.
2. To go away, as in seclusion, or to recuperate.
3. To go to bed.
4. To recede or disappear.
5. Shun contact with others.

Interestingly, he decided to keep working until he was well into his
70s. Despite the difficulties with the term, I will use 'retirement'
to refer to this transition from paid work.

Society has a nasty habit of demonising those who don't or can't
work. According to those who frame growing older negatively,
older people are a burden. If you are no longer working, you are

not contributing economically, and if you are a pensioner, you are also likely to be costing the rest of us money. This is based on the very narrow economic view of the world that we considered in chapter 2. As we'll see, people in later life contribute in lots of other ways: caring for partners, spouses or other family members with health conditions or disabilities; providing childcare for grandchildren; volunteering in a wide range of roles; and keeping community activities going. Such activities are often undervalued by society, because they don't generate direct economic contributions in the form of taxes, and yet they generate social value.

As I described in chapter 1, there have been phenomenal gains in life expectancy over the past 200 years – an increase of three years every decade. Lynda Gratton and Andrew Scott, the authors of *The 100-Year Life*, put this another way. They suggest these increases are equivalent to an extra six to eight hours every day.[2] They contend that if you had that much extra time you wouldn't just sleep through it, nor would you work a longer day. You would probably restructure your time. Perhaps eat more than three meals a day, take more breaks, have a nap, take up new hobbies. They explore how we might restructure our lives in response to longevity. So how can we help people make the most of this time? And how can society as a whole benefit?

In this chapter we'll look at people's experience of retirement and whether, and how, people can prepare for it. We'll consider both the benefits to individuals and society of volunteering by people in later life and what needs to change to enable more people to contribute if they wish to. We'll also look at the importance of carers and some of the challenges they face. What support do they get? What would be the implications for long-term care if these carers weren't available? The chapter concludes with some ideas for how to enable more people to be more active and for longer. We start by looking at people's views and experiences of retirement.

EXPERIENCES OF RETIREMENT

In Japanese, there is no word for 'retire', as in leave work for good, perhaps because many people strongly feel that being in work gives them purpose. *Ikigai* literally means 'life that is worthwhile' and, more generally, the happiness of always being busy.[3] It makes clear that we can get this purpose from paid work by pursuing a profession (something we're good at) or a vocation (something the world needs). We can also get this same sense of *ikigai* if we do things that are our passion (something we enjoy or are good at), such as a hobby, pastime or leisure activity, or our mission (something we believe in or can do for others) – perhaps a community activity, volunteering or helping someone else. This doesn't seem to be something unique to the Japanese. One of the key indicators of high wellbeing is feeling like you are *doing something worthwhile*.[4]

For many, retirement from paid employment is something to look forward to, but for others retirement can pose many challenges, and they find it difficult to adjust to their new role and circumstances. A YouGov poll conducted on behalf of the Centre for Ageing Better and the Calouste Gulbenkian Foundation, a charity which aims to improve the quality of life for all throughout art, charity, science and education, found that only half of those who plan to retire in the next five years are looking forward to it, a third are concerned about feeling bored (33%) and missing their social connections from work (32%), and nearly a quarter (24%) worry about losing their sense of purpose once they retire.[5]

There are, however, many things people enjoy about retirement. In the same survey, people who had retired in the past five years were asked about their experiences. Many didn't miss anything about work and 62% reported feeling more relaxed, 41% had spent more time on their hobbies or had started new ones, and more than 20% had got more involved in their local community. Of those who were retired, 12% did identify a loss of purpose or a lack of something to do, but the thing that most people missed about work was other people, with 36% of retirees stating that they missed the social contact of work.

In the same survey, half of those who were planning to retire in the next five years were looking forward to taking up new hobbies or having more time for existing hobbies – this was broadly similar across different socio-economic groups. However, a larger proportion of those in the higher socio-economic groups (ABC1) than those in lower socio-economic groups (C2DE) were looking forward to being more physically active – 43% versus just 27%. Only 15% of those in C2DE groups were looking forward to getting more involved in their local community in retirement, compared to 27% in ABC1 groups.

It seems that despite the debate about an end to retirement and the idea, popular among middle-class professionals, that everyone is retiring gradually and developing a portfolio career, this is still a minority experience. The same YouGov poll also found that 45% of workers planning to retire in the next five years had made no plans to reduce their hours or change the way they work, effectively meaning they would face a 'cliff edge' retirement, where they are (mostly) in full-time employment one day and suddenly stop the next. Just over a third – 37% – had already made plans to gradually reduce their hours, 13% had moved jobs to prepare for retirement, while a further 12% had become self-employed or started their own business.

There can be devastating consequences if people stop work without having anything in place, particularly if retirement is 'involuntary' (for example, a compulsory redundancy that turns into early retirement). Those who retire voluntarily have the best mental wellbeing and highest rates of social engagement, while those who retire involuntarily have the poorest levels of wellbeing and social engagement, according to analysis of the English Longitudinal Study of Ageing (ELSA). There are also socio-economic differences in the type of retirement experience, so while half of those retiring involuntarily were in the poorest two-fifths of the population in the period prior to retirement, half of those retiring voluntarily were in the wealthiest two-fifths of the population.[6] Some people struggle with retirement because they lose the social connections they had through work, no longer have a reason to get up in the morning and miss the structure that a job provided. This can leave people socially isolated and depressed. Some people, like James, one of our worried and disconnected from the Later Life Study (see box on page 130), struggle.

JAMES' STORY

James felt he had lost his purpose after retiring from work as a long-distance HGV driver at the age of 71. He'd carried on working until that age to make more money (he had never saved into his occupational pension), and now relies on the state pension and a small amount of rental income from his own property, but doesn't have many outgoings. James misses getting out and feeling like he's doing something useful.

Going to the pub is James' main social activity as he lives away from family and friends don't drop by. He meets two friends there, although he feels they are better off than him, because they still live with their partners. He goes about once a week, but otherwise spends a lot of time at home since his wife died. He doesn't feel there's much to look forward to.

Many people derive significant meaning and purpose from their jobs. Work is part of our identity. This can particularly be the case for men, who, despite changes in gender roles and entitlements to shared parental leave, are still more likely than women to be in full-time work. This may be why there is some evidence that unemployment has a more damaging impact on men's mental health than women who are unemployed, beyond the financial impact.[7] For some women, other identities as mother or carer can operate alongside the work identity. Research on men and women's experiences of retirement found that even mothers who had held senior roles tended to stress that their work was of secondary importance to their family. Furthermore, people of both genders who held less traditional or more flexible views about gender found the transition to retirement easier,[8] so it's important that we think about the psychological impact of stopping work, and that people are supported to find meaning and purpose from activities outside work.

But the nature of retirement is changing. We are seeing the emergence of new forms of working in later life, such as partial retirement, bridge jobs (often part-time roles taken on after people leave career employment, but before they retire) and 'un-retirement' (when people return to work having already retired). These new ways of working have the potential to enable more people to adjust to retirement and feel positive about the transition from paid work.

Some people find this transition easy and many don't miss work. Others find it more difficult and struggle. Some people plan their retirement, but many people find themselves 'retired' without having given a thought to what they will do with their time. What can help people make the transition from paid work to retirement in a way that enables them to remain positive?

PREPARING FOR RETIREMENT

A review of evidence on the experience of the transition to retirement found that those who felt they had control over their retirement had more positive outcomes. The extent of control over retirement planning and the retirement process are influenced by how well off you are – if you suffer from ill health you feel even less in control.[9]

The majority of people are underprepared for retirement, other than some financial planning by those with savings. The YouGov survey mentioned earlier also revealed that more than half of those who had retired in the past five years had sought no advice or help to prepare them for retirement.

This lack of preparedness for retirement is perhaps not surprising. Few employers provide pre-retirement courses. Where it exists the most common area of support is around finances. Support on health and wellbeing, and careers and future working life, is less common.

And yet when employees were offered the opportunity to take time to consider their retirement plans and to think about the social and emotional aspects, people found this very beneficial. An evaluation of a number of group-based interventions aimed at building the resilience and emotional wellbeing of people over 50 found participants were positive about being helped to consider wider elements of the transition to retirement, in some cases using tools like mindfulness and cognitive behavioural therapy techniques. In qualitative interviews 6 and 12 months after completing these courses, people still felt they had made a difference. Although these were small pilots, this research showed that there are a number of people who could benefit from group-based resilience training pre-retirement. One of the key findings of this evaluation was the positive impact the courses had on psychosocial factors such as perceived resilience and confidence.[10] A further evaluation supported this, with improvements in wellbeing, self-kindness and attitudes to both ageing and retirement. This evaluation also showed that people felt they were more engaged with thinking about their future and more likely to take practical steps, such as talking to their line manager.[11]

There are some existing initiatives in other countries that support people to make this transition. In the US, Encore.org supports professionals nearing the end of their careers to use their experience to help a charitable organisation, while continuing to be paid at a reduced rate. Julia Randell-Khan, Senior Fellow with Encore.org and Visiting Scholar at the Stanford Center on Longevity, describes the model as a three-pronged approach, matching a retired person, a non-profit organisation and a corporate sponsor. She claims there are well-established benefits for the individual, who is contributing their skills, and for the non-profit, which benefits from the individual's skills and experience, with little to no investment. Julia has established the Encore Fellows programme in the UK and is expanding access to the scheme to wider socio-economic groups and different career transition scenarios.

Employers need to focus more on preparing people for the retirement transition by starting conversations about people's goals early and supporting them to think about how they want to use their time after they stop paid work. One way in which people get meaning and purpose when they retire is by volunteering.

DOING GOOD

Is there an army of do-gooders waiting to be recruited if only we could motivate people in later life to take up volunteering? In fact, many people already give time to voluntary and community activities, often motivated to help others or improve their community in some way. The National Council for Voluntary Organisations (NCVO) estimates, based on the Community Life Survey in 2017-2018, that over 20 million people volunteered through a club, group or organisation.[12] Around one third of the adult population of all ages are involved in regular formal volunteering and another third regularly make an informal contribution. Throughout their lives most people will spend at least some of their time involved in community activities of some kind – only around 10% of people never make a contribution.[13]

Age itself does not appear to be a significant factor in determining whether or not people contribute. In the 2018-2019 Community Life Survey nearly one in three (28%) of those aged 65-74 reported regular volunteering in formal roles. This dropped slightly to one in four (24%) for those aged 75 and above, but was similar to levels of volunteering at younger ages – 22% of those aged 50-64 and 19% of those aged 16-49 volunteered. Rates of informal volunteering – that is giving unpaid help as an individual to people who are not relatives – were generally higher (though may still be under-reported) with 33% of those aged 65-74 reporting that they volunteered in informal ways. Rates among those aged 75 and above were similar (33%) and somewhat higher than among those aged 16-49 (24%) and those aged 50-64 (26%).[14]

The stereotype of a volunteer is of a middle-aged or older white woman. Indeed, they still make up a large proportion of those who are formally volunteering and are what is called the 'civic core'.[15] Some groups of people in later life are underrepresented, particularly in formal volunteering roles. Health and socio-economic status, and to a lesser extent ethnicity, are much more significant in determining propensity to engage in formal volunteering (rather than age). Some of these factors also mean people are more or less likely to help others in more informal ways. The evidence demonstrates clearly that those in poorer health are less likely to volunteer, with 41% of people who reported their health as excellent volunteering, compared to just 9% of people who reported their health as poor. There's also a clear correlation between socio-economic status and formal volunteering, with only 13% of people in the poorest fifth of the population reporting that they volunteer, compared with 43% of the richest fifth.[16]

Policy and organisations tend to focus on participation in formal volunteering and civic roles, such as magistrates and school governors or sitting on the boards of charities. Less is known about, and so less attention is given to, the many small acts of kindness and other informal ways people help out in their communities, such as people supporting neighbours, friends or members of their community. Research in deprived communities has shown high levels of engagement in informal ways of contributing to communities by people in later life and identified barriers to engaging in formal voluntary roles.[17]

As well as this, there appear to be lower levels of formal volunteering among people from BAME communities (18%) compared to 23% among people who define their ethnicity as white.[18] Older people from BAME communities face significant barriers to participation outside their immediate communities, yet within deprived communities there are high levels of contribution among minority ethnic groups, particularly within faith-based organisations and informally among friends and neighbours. These 'in-community' contributions are rarely recognised as a form of contribution that qualifies and so may be under-reported in surveys which rely on self-reporting. In community research commissioned by the Centre for Ageing Better, we found that many people were reluctant to categorise things such as helping a neighbour with shopping as a contribution, instead thinking this was just 'what people do'.[19]

So why does it matter that some people in later life are not involved in volunteering or making a contribution to their community?

WHY VOLUNTEERING IN LATER LIFE MATTERS

Volunteering in later life matters because there's value to the person doing it. There is good evidence of benefits, including: increased quantity and quality of social connections; enhanced sense of purpose and self-esteem; and improved life satisfaction, happiness and wellbeing.[20] Where people in later life feel valued and appreciated in formal volunteering roles, this contributes to reduced depression, but not all the benefits sometimes claimed for volunteering are well evidenced. For example, it doesn't seem to protect against social isolation or frailty in later life.[21] While volunteering is correlated with better health, this appears to be largely because healthier people are much more likely to volunteer. Similarly, there is little evidence that volunteering leads to employment for people in later life – labour market conditions are a far more important determinant.[22]

There are economic and social benefits, too. Age UK has estimated the value of volunteering by people over 65 as worth £2.7 billion.[23] Think of all the organisations locally you know that wouldn't function without volunteers: charity shops, local community centres, youth clubs, faith groups, sports associations and clubs, gardening projects and allotment committees. And it's not limited to voluntary organisations – one in five volunteers are in public services like hospitals or schools, according to the 2017-2018 Time Well Spent survey by NCVO.[24]

Some people may say that any action by government to promote 'civil society' is a cynical ploy to replace paid services. And indeed, volunteers are keeping public services like local libraries and rural bus services running. For example, in 2014 Sheffield City Council gave up control of 16 of its 28 libraries, otherwise earmarked for closure, to charities who try to run the service with volunteers, and when Essex County Council cut bus routes on Canvey Island, a local charity, Wyvern Community Transport, stepped in to run the bus service. Arguably, these services should be funded by local councils, but this is not a reason to discourage voluntary action within and across public services. For example,

Helpforce volunteers are working alongside clinical staff in the NHS to provide additional care and support to patients, assisting with mealtimes, providing companionship, helping patients get more mobile and so on.

However, the traditional model of volunteering may not be sustainable, as the so-called civic core – mainly white, middle class and women – who contribute disproportionately are unlikely to be able to maintain the current level of voluntary and community activities that exist. The older population is becoming more ethnically diverse. Women are more likely to be working and working to older ages, and will have other commitments, for example, they bear the burden of caring responsibilities. And there is no guarantee that these contributions will be sustained in future; younger generations who fit the 'civic core' profile may not act in the same way. There is a real threat to the volunteers of the future if organisations do not radically change and attract a different profile of volunteers.

HOW TO MAKE VOLUNTEERING MORE INCLUSIVE

Waiting until people retire to recruit them as volunteers may be too late. The evidence demonstrates clearly that leaving the labour market is not a significant determinant of making a contribution.[25] Few people start volunteering at the point of retirement.[26] Analysis of data from the English Longitudinal Study on Ageing suggests that volunteering rates are only about five to six percentage points higher for men and women five years after they retire than they were in the five years before reaching retirement age.[27] To promote volunteering at earlier ages, employers could give people time out, including paid volunteer days, to enable people to explore voluntary activities outside their job and perhaps increase the number of days for those approaching retirement. The government could also offer tax breaks for giving time, akin to Gift Aid on financial donations and the value of goods donated for sale at charity shops.

Work coaches in Job Centres also could encourage voluntary and community activity among those out of work, and the benefits system should not penalise or limit the number of hours that people on benefits such as Carer's Allowance, Employment and Support Allowance or Jobseeker's Allowance can spend volunteering. It can increase confidence and physical and mental wellbeing, all of which are often factors in successful job outcomes, particularly for those who have been out of work for some time. Having said all that, any moves to make community or voluntary action a 'requirement' for the unemployed is likely to change the very nature of this activity and may diminish the benefits.

Volunteering is a lifelong habit. All the evidence points to the importance of cementing these habits as early as possible in our lives and sustaining them as we get older.[28] Other life changes, such as the onset of a new long-term condition, bereavement or moving to a new house, do affect people's motivations and abilities to contribute. They can act as a spur to becoming involved, but they can also trigger withdrawal as people feel unable to continue volunteering and, once broken, the habit of volunteering can be hard to return to.

The reasons why people stop volunteering, or don't volunteer in the first place, are similar to the reasons that people fall out of work and include caring responsibilities and health problems. Similar barriers exist, too, such as lack of (affordable) transport, accessible facilities, flexibility, digital exclusion and ageist attitudes. Many of the solutions that would enable more people to sustain their ability to contribute are similar to the practices employers need to adopt to enable people to stay in work (see chapter 4). Good volunteer management and good line management come down to good people management – ensuring people feel valued, that 'reasonable' adjustments are made, that opportunities and time commitments are flexible, and that the application process is inclusive and fair.[29]

Volunteering needs to be made easy. The barriers identified above need to be removed, for example, by funders meeting the transport costs for people with mobility difficulties. The government or other charitable funders should set up a fund similar to Access to Work that can pay for adjustments to enable someone with a disability to fulfil a volunteering role, for example, by providing specialist equipment.

Organisations that use volunteers also need to attract a greater diversity of older people by using diverse images and language, as well as thinking about where and how they recruit. Word of mouth is very important, but it can tend to reinforce the lack of diversity, with people approaching people 'like them'. It is also important that organisations understand why older people want to volunteer and tailor the volunteering tasks and how they will make the experience feel worthwhile accordingly. If organisations that have volunteers adhere to some key principles (see box on page 139), they will be able to avert a major loss in volunteers.

Finally, there is a need to redefine volunteering. Many people are put off by the formal requirements and regular responsibilities that some roles require. There is a need for policy, funders and voluntary organisations to value and recognise the informal contributions and consider how these can be encouraged and supported without formalising them. There is also a need to blur the boundaries between recipient and beneficiary. Many of the current models are often about older people being helped by nice young people! The approach of North London Cares and other similar organisations is to create fun opportunities for young professionals to meet their neighbours. They don't talk about volunteering and try to encourage a more reciprocal friendship between those who attend their range of social events.

If volunteering and contributing in other ways to our communities is both valuable to society and benefits the individual, we surely want to encourage and support as many people as possible to get involved. This means: starting the habit early; making it easier for people to sustain and return to involvement after life changing events; ensuring the opportunities to contribute are available equally to people in all communities and from all backgrounds; and ensuring that all organisations that engage volunteers and mobilise action in communities operate in ways that are inclusive and age-friendly.

AGE-FRIENDLY AND INCLUSIVE VOLUNTEERING PRINCIPLES

Flexible and responsive:

- It fits around my life
- If life changes, I can adjust my commitment
- I know how to get involved, what to do and how to stop

Enabled and supported:

- I receive practical help with access, expenses and any training I want and need
- I feel supported and know who I can turn to with any questions

Sociable and connected:

- I have opportunities to meet and spend time with people, including from different backgrounds and age groups
- It makes me feel part of something

Valued and appreciated:

- The value of my effort is recognised, and people let me know they appreciate it regularly
- I feel like people appreciate what I do

Meaningful and purposeful:

- The work I do means something to me and feels purposeful
- I feel that what I do is worthwhile

Makes good use of my strengths:

- It allows me to use my skills and experiences, and to learn new skills
- I feel like my experience is respected and valued

Source: K. Jopling and D. Jones, (2019), Age-friendly and inclusive volunteering: Review of community contributions in later life, Centre for Ageing Better and Office of Civil Society.

WHO CARES?

One in eight adults (around 6.5 million people) provide unpaid care – defined as help with personal care or domestic tasks needed because of disability – to a family member, friend or partner (of whatever age).[30] While we know that the 'peak ages' for caring are in your 50s and 60s, and that you're more likely to be a carer if you're a woman than a man, we don't know a great deal about how old the people caring for older adults are. One NHS survey has shown that more than half of respondents over 55 were caring for someone over the age of 75. For carers over 85, nearly 90% are helping someone over 75.[31] These figures are all approximate, however, because surveys rely on people identifying themselves as carers and many do not. The last census, in 2011, found that many carers, especially those in the older age brackets, had health needs of their own. In fact, 65% of carers between 60 and 94 had a long-term health problem or disability themselves.[32]

Most unpaid, informal care for older people is provided either by their adult children or by their spouses or partners (estimates suggest 85% of the 1.4 million older people with disabilities living in their own homes receive unpaid care from either a spouse or partner or adult child).[33] It is clear that due to the increasing numbers of people over the age of 85, there will be a significant increase in the number of people needing care (see chapter 7), but will there be partners and family members available and willing to care for them?

Specific projections suggest that demand for unpaid care for people aged 75 and over will increase considerably in future because of the narrowing gap in life expectancy for men and women.[34] This will mean that more men will survive to older ages to provide care for spouses or partners, but they themselves may also need care. However, care by children will still be the most important source of unpaid care in 2032, because the majority of the oldest (aged 85 and over) will be 'single' (either widowed, divorced or never partnered). But it is projected that the growth in the need for care by adult children will far outstrip the number of people willing and available to provide such care, as we will see in the chapter on care.

Family carers do an amazing job, but not without personal cost. There needs to be better support for family and unpaid carers who provide many hours of care and support for their loved ones. Better recognition of the needs of carers is needed by health services, to make sure their health isn't being overlooked and they're able to access services (often difficult if they can't leave their relative unattended). GPs should be identifying carers and the recent NHS Long-Term Plan proposed that in future GPs will be rewarded based on how carer-friendly they are. Carers also have a right to their own assessment under the Care Act 2014, but many people are not aware of this or do not self-identify as carers, and social services have limited capacity to do these assessments. The assessment considers the impact on the carer and, if there is a significant impact, they may fund a support plan. This might include, for example, respite care, help with transport costs or other practical help, such as gardening, to enable the person to continue with their caring responsibilities. Access to respite care needs to be improved to give carers a break, whether through access to funded short stays in a residential setting or shorter periods of support in the home to allow the carer to look after their own health and wellbeing, and prevent them from becoming isolated. As a society we also need to think about more informal ways of supporting carers of older adults. Babysitting is often informally arranged within communities. Does taking care of older family members need to be as easy?

The value of this unpaid care is difficult to quantify. Without it many people would not be able to live at home and many more people would be admitted to care homes or hospitals. This unpaid and often ignored army of older carers is providing the most personal and intimate care for their loved ones, often in very challenging circumstances. The personal cost to the carers is enormous and can impact negatively on their wellbeing, health and social connections. For many it also impacts their ability to work and therefore their own financial security. It affects them not only while they are a carer, but often for the rest of their lives: it is difficult to return to work after the person you have been caring for dies, and to rebuild confidence and social networks that were lost. Social care is already heavily rationed, as we will see in chapter 7, both on the basis of need and means tested. If those in mid and later life were not providing this care, the costs of social care would be many times what they are today. It is time we started valuing care as a society or we risk making the 'care gap' even wider.

Those who fear the age shift in our society perceive retirement as unproductive and time wasted, and older people as a burden. And yet, as we have seen, older people are contributing hugely through voluntary activity and caring. If we are to harness the time, talents and experience of those in later life for the benefit of our communities, we need to replace the negative definition of 'retirement' with a more positive concept like *ikigai*, which recognises that later life is a time when people can pursue their passions or a mission, so they feel they have value and purpose. I haven't looked at passions – the time people spend pursuing hobbies and interests, learning new skills or enjoying leisure activities – although it is common for people to take up a hobby when they stop paid work and these no doubt enhance people's personal wellbeing.

It is clear that for some people the transition from paid work into retirement is difficult. They don't feel useful or valued by society. This is particularly true for those who find themselves involuntarily retired, as a result of, for example, ill health or redundancy. People find themselves 'retired' without having thought about what they might do with their time and, as a result, they struggle to find meaning and purpose, and some people become socially isolated and unhappy. But this need not be the case. If we help people plan emotionally and practically for retirement, give them time to prepare and adjust to the transition, enable them to make a positive choice to stop work at a time they feel ready to, including supporting them to keep working longer if they wish to, we would see more people actively making the most of their extra time.

Older people are the mainstay of voluntary and community organisations; making up the 'civic core', but there is a risk that unless things change this civic core is under threat. As the older population becomes more diverse, volunteering needs to be more inclusive, enabling more older people from BAME, and low income, backgrounds to volunteer. It also needs to become more flexible and recognise the changing needs and circumstances of people in later life, so that issues like poor health, caring and bereavement don't stop people participating. This will require active support from employers to encourage volunteering before people retire and from employment support programmes for those who are not working. Voluntary organisations and funders also need to provide the support and adjustments to make volunteering opportunities inclusive, and incentives and funding from government are essential, too.

Many people find themselves caring for loved ones in later life. Without these unpaid family carers, the current social care crisis would be a whole lot worse. As fewer adult children are willing or available to care, the burden increasingly falls to partners and spouses who themselves are also in later life. Carers need to be valued and supported so they can do these vital roles without a huge detriment to their own health, wellbeing and financial security. Employers need to be playing their part, but government action is required to create the same rights and entitlements for carers of older relatives that have enabled women to take leave and return to work following the birth of a child. Health services and local authorities must also fulfil their duties to these carers and provide them with the support they need to sustain their caring responsibilities without paying too great a price personally.

Helping people plan for their potentially long years of retirement and enabling them to continue to contribute long after they stop paid work, whether by volunteering or caring for others, will require some radical changes to how we view and value these extra years. This begins by seeing people in later life as an asset and not a burden to society. As we have seen, our ability to contribute and make the most of later life is affected by our health. In the next chapter we look at whether, as we live longer lives, we are also living in better health.

6

Healthy, longer lives – is it all downhill from here?

'An ageing population has pushed the NHS and social care system to the brink of collapse, the health minister Norman Lamb has warned …'

Gerri Peev, *Daily Mail* (May 2013)[1]

Along with pensions, the rising cost of health services is seen as one of the biggest fiscal challenges faced by governments internationally. The rise in health spending is often blamed on the increase in the number of older people. What are the drivers of our ever-spiralling health care costs?

Are we not just getting older but sicker too? As we survive the big killers of the past, like heart disease, cancer and stroke, are we simply living longer with more long-term conditions? And what about the rise in obesity and other unhealthy behaviours? How will these impact on our health in later life? If living longer means we're going to spend more years living in poor health, it seems like a nightmare. But catastrophising is not the answer. There are solutions if we choose to act wisely now.

Headlines scream out about the 'epidemic' of dementia. Older patients are described as 'bed blockers' because they can't be discharged from hospital. Older patients have not one, not two, but often three chronic conditions, all being treated with different drugs and by different specialists. The NHS is under strain and creaking at the seams. The blame is often squarely put on the rapidly rising numbers of older people. Will the age shift result in the long-predicted collapse of the NHS as the doom-mongers predict?

As we look to the future, science is revealing more about the underlying causes of the diseases of old age. Investors are speculating on a cure for ageing. Will science provide us with the solutions or will the inequalities we see in how well we age simply increase? Many of these fears may be valid, even if framed incorrectly as the 'fault' of older people. In this chapter I'll look at the real reasons for the spiralling costs of health care and what we can do to ensure our extra years are lived in good health.

WILL THE AGE SHIFT BANKRUPT THE NHS?

Shallow analysis and a lack of understanding of what we could do differently can lead doom-mongers to claim the ageing population will make the NHS unsustainable. Many point to rising health care expenditure, above the rate of inflation, and the growing proportion of public finances that health care consumes.

There have been several scapegoats for the rise in health care spending. In the 1950s doctors were blamed for wasting resources and 'excesses'. Because the NHS was now 'free' to patients, doctors were accused of handing out drugs and treatments too freely. By the 1960s and 1970s, worries about the ageing population and rising public expectations were added to the list of reasons for this growth. The economic context also worsened with the oil crisis and questions got louder about the sustainability of publicly funded health services (particularly from pro-market opponents of state-funded and state-run health care). Today, the most common reason given for the rapidly rising spending on health care is the ageing population. Is this true? And will it push health and social care spending to unsustainable levels?

In its July 2018 Fiscal Sustainability Report, the Office for Budget Responsibility (OBR), an independent organisation that is responsible for reporting on the performance of the economy and public finances, estimated that expenditure on health care will rise from 7.6% of GDP in 2022-2023 to 13.8% of GDP in 2067-2068 and it said this will put significant pressure on public finances.[2] The 'problem' seems even worse because there have been reductions in other areas of spending, for example, in education and defence, while spending on the NHS has been 'protected'. Health care is therefore consuming a growing share of public expenditure with nearly one in five of every £1 of public spending going on the NHS.

In addition to the pressures on the NHS, there's also concern at the additional costs of social care. However, we spend a lot less on adult social care than health services: 1.1% of GDP and 7.1% of GDP respectively in 2017-2018. The OBR's long-term projections for adult social care expenditure estimate an increase from 1.3% of GDP in 2022-2023 to 2.0% of GDP in 2067-2068. As we'll see in the next chapter, this is probably too little and we do need to consider how we increase funding on social care.

If you look in detail at the OBR's rationale, demographic changes (increasing numbers of people at older ages together with increases in the population due to migration) are estimated to increase health spending by only about 1% per year. This compares to a long-term historic rate of increase in spending on the NHS of 4% per year, suggesting that other factors contribute more.

So here's a different view. Most economists and analysts now conclude that the age shift is *not* the main problem. Most analysis of growth in health care expenditure points to technology as the main culprit – that means medical innovations, such as new drugs and changes in treatment and care, which enable us to help more people with a wider range of diseases and disorders.

Professor Robert Evans, a leading Canadian health economist, calls claims that health care systems are unsustainable because of changing demography a 'zombie' idea – an argument that's intellectually dead but will not stay buried. He says, 'Use and costs are primarily driven NOT by changing age structure, but by *changing patterns of care use* – what is done to and for patients.'[3]

For him, it's the decisions that doctors make about treatment that's the primary cause.

In most sectors of the economy, technology brings down the costs of products and services. In health care, technological advances and medical innovations can often *increase* the costs of providing care. We're not seeing robots looking after people – in fact, new technology rarely substitutes for human care – but instead more specialist surgical procedures and new drug therapies require more highly trained and specialist staff, who are usually paid more to reflect their longer training.

As well as this, medical innovation often results in identifying new diseases and developing new treatments and new interventions for people who in the past were untreatable. While fewer of us drop dead with a heart attack thanks to statins and stents or die of a stroke, we survive only to develop cancer and dementia, and this has a multiplier effect on health care costs.

This is the conundrum of improved survival rates, which result in longer lives but do not eliminate our 'need' for health care. As we explore below, one way to address this would be if we could have more of those extra years living in good health.

There is no inevitability that the age shift will bankrupt the NHS. Contrary to the simplistic argument often put forward, it's clear that the impact of an ageing population in and of itself does not threaten sustainability of health services. It only accounts for modest growth in spending of about 1% per annum, which, if economic growth returns (even to a lower than the historic rate, which has averaged around 2.2% per year over the last 40 years[4]) and levels of taxation are maintained, should be affordable. This doesn't mean controlling the other drivers of health care expenditure growth will be easy, but they require different remedies. Falsely blaming higher levels of spending on the ageing population detracts from the important (but difficult) decisions about what treatments and how much medicine we want to pay for.

148

DO WE COST MORE AS WE GET OLDER?

The short answer is yes – but probably not for the reasons you might think and there are significant ways in which this spend could be reduced. Health care spending per capita is indeed on average higher for someone aged over 65 than it is for someone aged 30. We are more likely to have an illness and need treatment when we are older. And so, with the age shift, an increase in the absolute number of people over 65 will increase how much we will spend on health care in total. But for every extra year we live we don't necessarily add another year of high-cost health care. We are generally staying healthier for longer and therefore the costs of care shift to older ages.

In fact, if we look more closely, we see that that the costs of health care are in fact concentrated in the last years of life. The relationship observed between age and per capita health care expenditure is in fact due to proximity to death rather than age per se. The OBR agrees: the higher costs at older age are due to the 'fact that spending rises very sharply in the last year of life ("death-related costs")'. A wide range of studies in a range of countries, including the USA, the Netherlands, Switzerland and England, have all confirmed that age is a much less significant determinant of health care expenditures than proximity to death.[5] Nuffield Trust research found that, from the age of 60, social care costs at end of life increase and in-patient costs decrease. By the age of 90, end of life social care costs exceed in-patient hospital costs.[6] How close we are to dying – and therefore the need for care and intensity of treatment – is a big factor in how much is spent on our health and social care.

This is mainly due to choices about the intensity of treatment, and the application of new treatments and technologies in an attempt to stave off the inevitable – death. This opens up a debate about a radically different approach to end-of-life care and challenges our attitudes to death.

HAVE WE OVER MEDICALISED DEATH?

There is a prevailing value which determines decision-making among medical professionals – the rule of rescue. When there are choices about how we want to deploy scarce resources, priority is given to saving lives. As we've seen, our quest to defy death appears to result in an intensity of treatment in the last years and months of life. This can sometimes result in prolonged treatment at end of life. This is not only distressing for patients and their families, but costs more, too. If policy makers are serious about cost control, they need a relentless focus on end-of-life care. A focus on a good death could simply cost less.

Economists writing in a British Medical Association report in 1967 wrote that 'the concept of life as beyond price' is 'deeply ingrained in the public mind'. Consequently, 'It is only when the public is aware that everything is not, and cannot, be done to save and perpetuate their lives that they are likely to question the adequacy of the State's present provision.'[7] This fundamental issue of how much a life is worth – the price we are willing to pay to live as long as humanly possible – is at the heart of the dilemma.

Professor Sir Muir Gray, a leading public health doctor, told me how things have changed over his 50 years of clinical work. He has seen a shift from 'undertreatment of older people, due to ageism, to overtreatment of older people, due to lack of insight into what people want and the limitations of health care.' He went on to say, 'We're now thoughtlessly overusing it [medicine] without finding out what is really bothering the person.' Having conversations with patients and helping them with decision-making, including weighing up the risks and benefits, in advance of any treatment could make a difference.

There is growing interest in what is called shared decision-making, where doctors involve patients more actively in considering what they want and factor this into a joint decision about which treatment options to follow. Some doctors have adopted a different style of consultation and use decision aids such as videos or online tools to help people understand the options and elicit their goals and preferences. The NHS in Scotland has been implementing this approach since 2015 as part of what it calls 'realistic medicine'. In Wales this approach is called 'prudent health care'. This has similar principles, including 'Do only what is needed – no more, no less', and the public, patients and professionals are viewed as equal partners. The NHS in England is now rolling out shared decision-making across the country as part of what it calls 'universal personalised care'. However, particularly when it comes to end-of-life treatments, these are difficult conversations to have for professionals, the individuals affected and their families.

Death is one certainty we can plan for, and yet many of us do not have a will and have not set up a power of attorney or advance directive setting out our wishes for when we are no longer able to make informed decisions for ourselves. There are often extremely difficult trade-offs to be made about quality and length of life. These are powerfully illustrated by Atul Gawande, a US surgeon, who tells the story of his own father's care and death from cancer in his bestselling book *Being Mortal*. He asks his father what trade-offs he would be willing to make. He shares the example of another patient who'd said if he were able to watch football on television and eat chocolate ice cream then that would be good enough for him. His own father felt that being around other people was most important and having some control over his life. Later in the book, after his father has had surgery on the tumour and decided not to have chemotherapy, he recalls a conversation between a palliative care nurse and his father. At this stage in his illness, he wanted to be free of pain and happy and valued being able to type so he could use email and Skype to connect with family and friends all over the world.[8] I had a similar conversation with my own father after he had drawn up an advance health directive, albeit at a time when he was in good health, with no immediate prospect of death. He said that as long as he is still enjoying watching Manchester United playing football on TV then he would want to live and treatment to continue. Clearly, where care and treatment options to prolong life are available, it is difficult to weigh these up against the expected negative impact on quality of life.

To reduce the risk of decisions made without informed patient consent, advance directives, otherwise known as advance decision statements or living wills, can be drawn up. These set out your wishes to refuse certain treatments under certain circumstances, so that if you are unable to communicate, health professionals and family members can act on these.

In the case of my father-in-law, there was no such written information. He collapsed at home early one morning. My mother-in-law heard him fall, but couldn't get to him, because he had fallen against the living room door. She called an ambulance and the police also attended to assist. Once the paramedics could get to him, they attempted to resuscitate him. They were able to get a pulse and made a decision to transfer him to a specialist cardiac unit where his condition could be assessed. The ambulance took him to hospital, where he spent his last four days in an induced coma and on life support. This then left the family to make the difficult decision to withdraw life support on the advice of doctors when it was clear that he was effectively brain dead. Looking back, it is hard to see how different decisions could have been made. It would have been difficult for the family and the paramedics to have taken a decision on the spot not to resuscitate. My father-in-law had not discussed his wishes with anyone and there was no do not resuscitate order. The paramedics did not know how long his heart had stopped for and therefore the extent of the brain damage.

The fact is that only around 2 out of 10 people who are resuscitated in hospital survive and leave hospital, and the survival rates in other settings are even lower,[9] yet at every step things are geared towards intervention, even when survival is unlikely. A more fundamental change in the approach to end-of-life care is needed if we are to reduce this overtreatment.

DYING WELL

Often people are only offered palliative care (meaning access to specialist nursing, hospice care or care at home to prepare for end of life, including pain relief if needed) when all medical options are exhausted, but research shows it might be beneficial to consider this option earlier. One study found that patients with terminal cancer and end-stage heart failure lived on average 29 days longer in hospice care. There was not, however, any difference for breast or prostate cancer patients.[10] Another study of patients with a type of lung cancer found that patients who had been offered early palliative care were less likely to receive aggressive treatments, but had higher quality of life and mood scores, and on average survived longer.[11] Switching to palliative care earlier could reduce medical intervention, save money and improve quality of life for the time people have left.

If people are to have a different (and less medical) death, it means that those caring for them need to have the right training and support, whether they are professional carers or family members. Many care home staff feel unsupported or they may not feel they have the equipment or nursing staff to deal safely with residents who become very ill. When a resident's condition deteriorates this often means they call 999 and send the person to A&E, even though this may not be the best course of action for the patient if they are near the end of life. This often means that people die in hospital rather than in a care home or at home. A number of pilots have been running in England to give better medical support to care homes. A recent evaluation of one scheme in Nottinghamshire found a 23% reduction in emergency admissions compared to similar residents in other parts of the country.[12]

If more residents of care homes are to die there (the average length of stay is around 26 months before people pass away[13]), care homes need to be more like hospices. This is a far cry from what most care homes currently are (or are funded to be). Care homes should embrace the hospice philosophy and ethos of active pain management and ensuring dignity and a good death. This will require investment. Training needs to be given to care home staff to give them the confidence to help people at the end of life. They need to be supported on the premises by district nurses and GPs, and have access to, and the confidence to use, stronger pain medication, as is the case in hospices.

As well as health and care staff, family members need support to feel more confident about caring for people at the end of life. Most of us have not seen someone die and, as the tradition of an open coffin being laid out at home is rare these days, few of us have even seen a dead body. Many people want to die at home, but are not able to do so, perhaps because the family are afraid of the responsibility and what this might entail. To help, there are increasing numbers of people training as end of life or death doulas, who provide support in the final months, weeks and days, attending to the individual and family's practical, emotional and spiritual needs alongside medical care. They help people to live life meaningfully right to the end. Other schemes, such as the Marie Curie Helper service, play a similar role in providing support and companionship to people in their own homes at end of life. If we are to de-medicalise death, then people need to be supported to remain at home and families helped by others in their community who may be able to guide them through.

These actions would go some way to reducing the sometimes intrusive, unwanted, ineffective and even harmful medical care that is given to people at end of life. Many people want more control over how and when they die. The vast majority of people say they want to die at home. According to a Dying Matters survey in 2009, more than 70% of us want to die at home, with only 7% thinking a hospital would be the best place to die. And yet more than 60% of people currently die in hospital. Although just under a quarter (23%) of people thought being pain free was the most important thing for end-of-life care, and another quarter prioritised keeping their dignity, slightly more people thought that being with friends and family was the most important thing in end-of-life care (25%).[14]

Dying well will require health and social care to change the approach to end of life, to find ways of making it more acceptable to withhold treatment, and to support families to have difficult conversations. Earlier conversations and access to palliative care would help people to make a positive choice and to prioritise quality of life over extension of life.

LET'S TALK ABOUT DEATH

It's tempting just to say to a family member, 'I hope someone will give me a pill when the time comes,' as my grandma said to us. She didn't want to be a burden on anyone. But when would have been the right time to do this, who would have administered the pill and where would they have sourced the lethal medicine from? As it was, Grandma died in hospital having got bladder cancer at 93. Despite her wishes to die in the care home, when she fell ill the staff called an ambulance and she was admitted to hospital. What are we supposed to do when those we love tell us that they would actively want their life to end when their quality of life reaches a certain point? Currently in the UK any such actions would bring criminal charges.

The debate about voluntary euthanasia, while rejected again in 2016 by a parliamentary vote in both the Commons and the Lords, will inevitably return. A generation who have been used to a great deal of choice and personal autonomy, who may have seen their own parents suffering with dementia or having a severely diminished quality of life at the end, may want to choose something different for themselves. Those who can afford to do so might travel to clinics in places where assisted death is legal, such as Switzerland. Others could take things into their own hands and commit suicide (if they are able). It is vital we have a full and open debate about whether as a society we want to legalise assisted suicide or voluntary euthanasia.

We also need a more balanced debate about decisions on the compassionate withdrawal of treatment, as well as the appropriate levels of pain management without fear of criminal charges. Doctors are often concerned about increasing pain medication or withdrawing feeding when someone is dying due to fears of litigation and criminal charges. The case of Harold Shipman, a GP who was convicted of murdering 15 patients but who may have killed over 200 mostly elderly patients by giving them strong painkillers, may explain doctors' reluctance and fear of administering strong pain medications to patients. In a confusing and contradictory mix of stories where children are 'denied' expensive medicines for the treatment of rare diseases, while people in vegetative states are kept alive and on feeding tubes, it's hard to know which set of values should take precedence. Is the ideal to be kept alive at any cost, emotional or monetary? Or to die a dignified death without over-treatment? And according to whose wishes – next of kin or the medics? Whatever the conclusion of that debate it is vital that everyone has the opportunity to live a full life to the end and to be supported to have a good death. This is the philosophy that underpins palliative care.

Do societal attitudes to death and dying need to be challenged more generally? This is the idea behind death cafés (see box on page 157). I recently attended one near where I live and found myself sitting at a table with a group of people of all ages. We discussed the challenges of caring for someone who is dying, feelings of grief and how to cope with bereavement, the challenge of writing a will, organising a funeral and clearing your house if you have no partner or children. The reasons people came and the things they wanted to talk about were many and varied. It felt strangely normal to have this conversation and increasingly I find myself chatting more to friends about their own and their parent's wishes and funeral plans – and not feeling this a morbid conversation, but the stuff of life.

DEATH CAFÉS

Death cafés are meetings hosted by individuals, often in a café or with tea and cake, for people to talk freely about death. Conversation can be aided by a volunteer host but is led by the group as a whole. Since the first death café was held in London in 2011, hosted by a Buddhist by the name of Jon Underwood, hundreds of meetings have been held globally, some as a one-off and others on a regular basis.

Anyone can host a death café. The aim isn't necessarily to talk about bereavement but dying and death in general. Some groups are specific to the experience of death and dying in certain communities, like death cafés specifically for the LGBT community, but the main purpose is to provide a place where talking about death and dying is welcomed, rather than uncomfortable. While conversation is unstructured, the concept of a good death or what songs you might like at your funeral or how you would like to be remembered may well be covered.

It is perhaps time we accepted we are mortal. While we maintain this social taboo and avoid all talk of death, not only does fear of death overshadow an individual's later years, but the conspiracy of silence can result in over-treatment and poor decisions. Facing up to death as the one certainty in life opens up the possibility of having conversations and planning ahead, which might give us a higher chance of a good death when it comes. But what about living well? We saw in chapter 1 that we are living longer on average, so let's look at whether we are living longer, healthier lives or getting sicker as we get older.

ARE WE GETTING SICKER?

In the 1970s the idea of the 'epidemiological transition' was put forward. It posited that while public health measures introduced in the late 19th and early 20th century together with new medical discoveries were contributing to a decline in infectious diseases, these were being replaced by a new challenge – so called 'degenerative and man-made' diseases or what we would now call chronic diseases or long-term conditions.[15] The rise of chronic diseases was recognised as posing challenges in a British Medical Association report of 1967: 'They [chronic illnesses] do not lend themselves to immediate medical success nor threaten immediate death but require costly and repetitive medical servicing of faulty bodies.'[16] Chronic conditions like Type 2 diabetes are particularly common at older ages.[17] The statistics show that the prevalence of chronic conditions rises with age, so that by the age of 65 16% of people have three or more chronic or long-term conditions.[18] This multi-morbidity – people having several different diseases – feeds into another issue – polypharmacy – taking multiple drugs at the same time, which can often interact with each other.

James, one of the worried and disconnected group from the Later Life Study, is typical of this sort of patient. He has a number of long-term health conditions, including Type 2 diabetes, atrial fibrillation, dizzy spells and memory loss. Although he takes the medication the doctor prescribes him, James doesn't pay much attention to what he eats and drinks, and isn't particularly active. However, he is glad that a preventative approach has been taken to his memory loss. Although James doesn't always think the activities in his cognitive stimulation course are helpful, he is relieved that his memory loss is being tackled, as he has recently lost his wife to dementia and is wary of going through the same thing.

While medical advances have been successful at stopping people dying early (as we have seen in chapter 1), this has resulted in more people living in poor health for longer. Until recently, rises in life expectancy were matched by rises in healthy life expectancy, i.e. the period of life lived in ill health stayed the same. But healthy life expectancy is now rising at a slower pace than overall life expectancy. As the chart below shows, in 2009-2011 women were expected to live 82.4 years of which 63.8 were

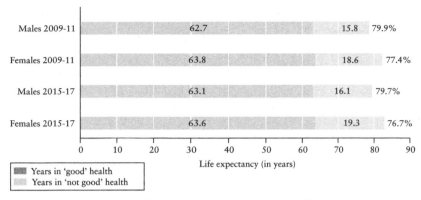

Males 2009-11 — 62.7 — 15.8 — 79.9%

Females 2009-11 — 63.8 — 18.6 — 77.4%

Males 2015-17 — 63.1 — 16.1 — 79.7%

Females 2015-17 — 63.6 — 19.3 — 76.7%

Life expectancy (in years)

■ Years in 'good' health
░ Years in 'not good' health

Healthy life expectancy at birth, and the proportion of life spent in 'good health' by sex.
Source: Office of National Statistics, *Health state life expectancies, UK: 2015 to 2017* (2018).

in good health. While life expectancy increased in 2015-2017 to 82.9, equivalent to an additional six months, just over two of those additional months were in good health.[19]

It is now widely known that there is a 15-year difference in life expectancy between people in the poorest areas and the richest areas.[20] A similar gap exists for healthy life expectancy. Men living in the most deprived areas of the UK spend 18.3 fewer years in good health than men in the least deprived areas. For women, the gap is 19.8-years.[21] This means that people living in areas like Kensington and Chelsea in London can enjoy, on average, 18 more years of good health compared to people in places like Blackpool or Manchester. This is a scandal and has far-reaching implications, for example early onset of disability means people falling out of work before state pension age (an issue we looked at in chapter 4) and because of the poor housing conditions people are often living in they will experience these conditions as more disabling than those living in richer areas with the same condition. It is vital we address the causes of these inequalities from cradle to grave. Michael Marmot, Director of University College London's Institute of Health Equity, has led research on health inequalities for more than 40 years, including a strategic review of health inequalities in England post-2010. In this report, he highlighted how issues such as tackling childhood poverty and improving educational attainment, improving the quality of work and increasing pay and progression will all impact on later life health outcomes.[22]

The reality is that those of us who are educated and reasonably well off enjoy not only longer lives, but also live longer in good health than people on lower incomes. There are growing inequalities in the experience of ageing.

Much of the burden of ill health we see at older ages is not an inevitable fact of ageing. Much of it is actually a result of cumulative disadvantage over the life course. The impact of external stressors on the body accumulates over a lifetime and this is partly why we see earlier onset of disease in the most disadvantaged, who have been exposed to more risk factors and stressors, and often from an earlier age. For example, smoking is more common among people in lower socio-economic groups, children living in more deprived areas are exposed to higher levels of air pollution, and studies have shown a link between inequalities and stress levels.[23] When we experience stress our bodies go into fight or flight mode, which produces higher levels of cortisol. If we experience chronic stress, these levels remain high and increase the risk of many health problems. Longitudinal research has found that socio-economic status in early life continues to impact on health outcomes in later life.[24]

Dr John Beard, former Director of Ageing and Life Course at the World Health Organisation, thinks that these differences are a huge challenge to society: 'In older age groups there is incredible diversity ... Where you sit on the spectrum, both in terms of health and resources, is not random, it is very heavily driven by the cumulative impact of advantage and disadvantage. People at the top in good health are also the people who live in good circumstances, they are the beneficiaries of the cumulative impact of advantage. People at the bottom bear the impact of cumulative disadvantage. This means that they also have greatest needs and the least resources to draw on. In setting policy, we must not reinforce those inequities. We should not just be thinking about raising the average wellbeing of older people, we must give particular attention to those at the bottom, so we can raise their rate disproportionately to the rich and narrow the gap.'

Although on average we are living longer, we are living more of those years not in good health. Is this going to push health services to breaking point?

PRESSURE ON SERVICES AND A BROKEN MODEL OF CARE

Every day we hear about the problems of the NHS: people waiting for hours on trolleys in corridors; ambulances queuing up outside A&E departments; not enough staff to care for the rising number of frail older patients; and 'bed blockers' unable to leave hospital due to the lack of availability of social care to support them at home or too few beds in care homes.

But pressure on services in recent years is less to do with the ageing population per se and more to do with the financial crisis and austerity, which has resulted in a historically low period of flat real-terms growth for the health service, just 1.3% between 2009 and 2016 compared to an average of 4.1% per annum between 1955 and 2009.[25] Some of the pressure has been absorbed through pay restraint and so-called efficiency measures (delivering the same care for less), but the other pressures from new technology continue apace. The only ways to manage these when faced with a fixed budget are for waiting times to rise, quality to fall or care to be denied (commonly known as rationing).

Within the NHS there is a misallocation of resources. Most of the money and services are focused on acute care in hospitals. The majority of bed days in hospital are taken up by patients with chronic conditions, admitted with problems such as renal failure as a result of complications from Type 2 diabetes as well as urinary tract infections. These lengthy stays in hospital are due to a lack of suitable alternative care settings. More NHS resources need to be spent on enabling people to manage their health conditions and prevent acute exacerbations – to understand when and why they might get a urinary tract infection and treat it earlier, for example. This requires more proactive care in the community or home and active rehabilitation to enable people to function as well as they did before they got ill.

John Beard, the public health expert I spoke to, agreed that the role of health care services should be to increase and maintain people's functionality, noting that, 'Most health systems evolved to cure acute conditions, initially trauma and infectious diseases. They are very poorly designed to meet the needs of older people with chronic conditions and multi-morbidities. Most health systems react to the presentation of individual conditions and treat them. They monitor their impact in terms of that condition, rather than the broader benefit to the individual or the interaction between conditions. Health care systems need to be designed so services are integrated around the whole older person and their aspirations and deliver what is needed to help them meet those aspirations.' He went on to say, 'We have very medically dominated health systems, where decision-making often centres on the doctor with other staff implementing these choices. We need to challenge this and become much more multi-disciplinary and extend beyond traditional health care to include social and community care. An ideal system would span multiple disciplines and break down silos but would also move beyond the health domain and be framed around the aspirations of the older person themselves.'

The NHS fails to live up to this ideal, in common with many health systems worldwide. While the individual medical treatment for a particular disease can be world-class, for elderly patients with multiple conditions it feels fragmented, impersonal and often fails to improve the quality of life. There have been efforts in recent years to integrate care, by bringing together teams across hospital and community health care and pooling some funding between health and social care through the Better Care Fund. However, cuts in social care and community health services have undermined these efforts. Older people with higher levels of dependency cannot be discharged home because packages of care and support are not in place, resulting in longer stays in hospital. While the woes of the NHS are often blamed on the rising numbers of older people, the reality is that many of these patients require social care, not medical care. As we'll see in the next chapter, we need to both increase the amount of funding for social care and look at new models of providing care. But there also needs to be a shift within health care from a focus on treating disease to a greater focus on preventing these diseases in the first place.

A RADICAL APPROACH TO PREVENTION OF DISEASE

It would be hard to miss the fact that as a nation, our waistlines have expanded and our sofa-time increased. Unhealthy behaviours such as smoking, drinking, lack of exercise and overeating mean high rates of chronic conditions and incidence of cancer. According to the Global Burden of Disease Study, which measures the leading causes of disease, the biggest risk factors of ill health are smoking, poor diet and high body mass index (i.e. being overweight or obese).[26]

What we need is a radical approach to prevention to reduce the incidence of chronic diseases. This will require tackling the main causes of ill health – smoking, alcohol consumption, lack of physical activity and obesity. Too often these are seen as being matters of personal responsibility, of individual choice and lifestyle, but the fact is that for most people these behaviours are not rational choices. Smoking is an addiction. For some people alcohol is, too, but for many more it is seen as a socially acceptable drug. For people on lower incomes, access to affordable healthy food is more limited, since it is usually more expensive. Agricultural and food subsidies mean that foods that are high in sugar and animal fat are cheaper than fresh fruit and vegetables. We are likely to be more physically active if we have access to good public transport.[27] It doesn't just depend on whether someone is motivated and can afford to go to the gym. There is strong evidence that changing the environment around us and effectively reducing choice, or at least not relying solely on people's own 'willpower' to change, reduces harmful health behaviours.[28] If there's less sugar in fizzy pop, we will consume less when we buy a can!

Professor Sir Muir Gray, the leading public health doctor I mentioned earlier, has been trying to get people to be more active for many years: 'Very rarely do I try to motivate people, because people mostly want to do the right thing, so it is better to identify the barriers to activity and work to reduce those barriers.' If walking to the shops isn't possible because there's no pavement in your village, that's a barrier that will stop people going out and moving around. In a recent article in *The Lancet*, Theresa Marteau, Director of the Behaviour and Health Research Unit at the University of Cambridge, and other leading health researchers argued that two complementary approaches to disease prevention are needed: targeting individuals at high risk and targeting whole populations. They go on to write, 'Targeting individuals through, for example, weight loss programmes without changing the environments that promote excessive energy consumption is akin to treating people for cholera and then sending them back to communities with contaminated water supplies.'[29]

Take smoking, for example: smoking rates are falling among younger age groups, but there are still persistent smokers in their 50s and 60s, particularly among lower socio-economic groups. These inequalities in smoking rates among those in mid-life and onwards will contribute to continued inequalities in both how long and how well people live into old age. The recent NHS Long Term Plan, outlining priorities for the next 10 years, has committed to investing in a more intense programme of support for smokers known as the Ottawa Model. This identifies people who smoke on admission to hospital and provides them with advice, dedicated counselling and follow-up after discharge. It will be offered to those who are admitted to hospital and long-term users of mental health services, as well as people with learning disabilities. This is based on evidence that low-income smokers could benefit from more intensive interventions to reach the same levels of quitting as high-income smokers. Other smoking cessation support is funded by local authorities and has been cut back since public health funding was transferred from the NHS in 2013.

However, this needs to be accompanied by further measures to tackle smoking at a population level. Reductions in smoking rates and harms have been achieved with the introduction of a series of measures, including a ban on smoking in public places, extending the ban to cars where there are children present, introduction of plain packaging and high levels of taxation on tobacco. Between 2000 and 2016, smoking rates amongst adults over 16 reduced by 10 percentage points.[30] Would a more radical step be to eliminate tobacco smoking completely? It is perhaps not impossible to imagine a complete ban on tobacco products, given the societal shift we have seen since the smoking ban and the widespread marketing of nicotine alternatives through e-cigarettes. Other steps might include raising the legal age, increasing tax on hand-rolled tobacco and better publicity for smoking cessation services targeted at those most likely to smoke.

Alcohol consumption rates have generally been decreasing, except among the over 55s. Since 2012, the 55–64 age group has had the highest levels of drinking.[31] While the Royal College of Psychiatrists says some of the increase in the percentage of those with alcohol dependency who are over 65 can be explained by demographic changes (there are more people over 65, so they make up a greater proportion of the people with alcohol dependency), most evidence suggests that older people are more likely to drink little, but often.[32] According to the Office of National Statistics, 18% of those over 65 had consumed alcohol at least five days in the last week, compared to 2% of those 16-24, but only 6% of those had more than 8 units (for men) and 6 units (for women) on their heaviest drinking day in the last week, compared to 20% of those 16-24.[33] Despite this, nearly half (46%) of hospital admissions that are either primarily or secondarily attributable to alcohol are among patients age 55–74.[34]

If successful, projects that specifically target older drinkers could contribute to reduced alcohol consumption at older ages. Drink Wise, Age Well, which is currently being piloted in five local areas across the UK, offers individual support to help people think about how their drinking is affecting their lives, via home visits, group sessions and social activities. It also provides more general advice around drinking and age and is trying to raise awareness around the way alcohol metabolises in your body as you get older, and how it can affect everyday life, as well as your later life. The aim is to help people make healthier choices about alcohol as they age. This project is still at a pilot stage and there are no plans as yet to roll it out nationally.[35]

Such targeted education programmes alone are unlikely to bring about a major reduction in alcohol consumption among older adults. Heavier regulation of where and when alcohol is sold, restrictions on advertising and sponsorship, and further price incentives, such as minimum unit pricing, could make a difference, but such policies are unlikely to prove publicly acceptable without a major shift in attitudes, norms and habits when it comes to regular drinking, particularly among older generations.

Around 60% of the adult population in the UK are overweight or obese.[36] The rise in obesity is likely to increase the prevalence of diabetes, heart disease and stroke. Projections suggest that this could result in increased expenditure of £1.9-2 billion per year by 2030.[37] Dr Zoe Wyrko, the consultant geriatrician behind Channel 4's *Old People's Home for 4 Year Olds*, was pretty matter of fact about the likely impact of obesity when I asked her how it impacts on people's health in later life. She said, 'I don't see them. They don't get to me. They don't live into deep old age.' The stark truth is that people with clinical or morbid obesity experience many complex issues. As a geriatrician, Wyrko is being called on to look after severely obese people in their 50s, because they have complex health and care needs, predominantly driven by their obesity, that are usually only seen in older people. They need the skills and multidisciplinary approach that geriatricians specialise in. Tackling obesity has to be a major priority.

While intense programmes such as the NHS-funded Type 2 Diabetes Prevention Programme are part of the solution, more radical changes are needed to change the make-up of our food by regulating the food and drinks industry to reduce sugar, calorie content and portion sizes. The introduction of the levy on soft drinks in the UK (the 'sugar tax') in 2018 has encouraged the producers of soft drinks to take a significant number of calories out of the food chain. They would otherwise have had to pay the tax (or pass it on to consumers) if they had continued to have such high levels of sugar in their products. To avoid paying, most producers took the option of 'reformulating' the drinks and taking some sugar out, so people are consuming less sugar even if they're buying the same amount of pop. Mexico saw around a 7% reduction in the purchase of sugary soft drinks after producers were forced to increase the price by 10%.[38] This has the potential to reduce obesity and its associated illnesses over the long term.

The Chief Medical Officer has produced guidelines based on evidence of how much physical activity an adult should do to get health benefits. This recommends that adults should take part in at least 150 minutes of moderate intensity physical activity a week. And yet most of us are not achieving this. Women do moderately worse than men and the rates decline with age. Less than 51% of men and 42% of women over the age of 65 are doing the recommended physical activity levels.[39]

Getting more physical activity is not just about finding time to do sport or exercise, it requires a shift in society to get us all moving more. Professor Sir Muir Gray blames the loss of fitness at older ages on 'decades of sitting down, not to laziness'. He argues, 'It's an environmental problem' as a result of more people driving, more people in office jobs and areas with no green space to run around in. Marketing like the adverts by Sport England that 'This Girl Can' has limited impact on rates of physical activity. There is also not strong evidence showing that 'exercise on prescription', in which individuals are targeted with free or subsidised access to gyms, has a long-term effect on behaviour change.[40].

To increase physical activity across the population, we need to redesign the environment. The decline in manual work and the rise in office-based work means we are generally more sedentary than in the past and if you rely on a car to get around, you will also be more sedentary than someone who uses public transport. The health benefits of fads like standing desks are not yet proven, but other actions that reduce the sedentary nature of much work by promoting more physical activity during the day or on the commute to and from work should help. While older generations grew up in an era before the car and were used to walking greater distances, today many places are not designed to encourage people to be active every day. To counter this will require investment in active transport policies to encourage cycling, to make streets more walkable by fixing paving and making sure they are well lit, and ensuring green spaces are safe and accessible to everyone.

There's rightly a lot of focus on physical health, but the mental health of older people is equally important and yet often neglected by health professionals. One in five people in the UK aged over 16 showed symptoms of anxiety or depression in 2016.[41] Similar rates are recorded among those aged 65 or over (22% and 28% of men and women respectively)[42] and yet 85% of older people with depression or anxiety receive no help at all from NHS.[43]

There's significant underdiagnosis of this problem and many older people with symptoms are not getting treatment. Older people who are diagnosed are less likely to be referred for talking therapies than younger people. It is vital older people get equal access to the full range of treatments for anxiety and depression. Access to psychosocial support, such as mindfulness, as people approach retirement has been shown to improve confidence, and help people feel better able to manage the transition between work and retirement. This association was particularly strong in people who had low confidence prior to attending the pre-retirement courses.[44]

Boosting healthy ageing through a committed new focus on prevention will not only reduce the costs of health and social care but will also result in higher productivity (as we saw in the chapter on work, poor health is a leading reason for people leaving work early).

Public health and the NHS have focused in recent decades on preventing premature death. Earlier diagnosis, the widespread prescription of statins and hypertensives to prevent strokes and heart disease, and more rapid access to cancer treatment have resulted in lower mortality rates and improved life expectancy, but we now need to shift the focus to maximising the time lived in *good* health. This will require as much focus on prevention as treatment. I've looked at changes we can make now to address the causes of ill health, but some think that in the not-too-distant future we may be able to treat 'ageing' itself.

THE PROMISE OF A CURE FOR AGEING

Are the diseases of old age inevitable? No. It's a surprise to some to understand that ill health and disability are not an inevitable part of ageing. Our chronological age is associated with a higher prevalence of many diseases, but there is huge variability in health status among people of the same age. Most disease is caused by a combination of genetics, lifestyle and environmental factors. Chronological age is therefore not a useful indicator of someone's health, fitness or capability. Recent scientific developments can shed some light on why this is and offer some suggestions as to where the solutions might lie.

Biologically speaking, ageing begins at 30 or even earlier. Things do go wrong and things wear out. This process is called senescence, and it refers to the decline in organ and cell function that occurs from repeated use. To oversimplify, if you imagine the body as a machine, the more it's used the more worn the cogs become, but a well-oiled engine and one that is regularly serviced will last longer than one that has had no maintenance.

Science is giving us a new perspective on ageing – at the cellular level. Telomeres are the end sections of DNA, at the end of our chromosomes, and telomeres shorten as we age. This shortening is one of the biological pathways towards disease. In their book *The Telomere Effect*, biologist Elizabeth Blackburn and psychiatrist Elissa Epel use the metaphor of shoelace tips. The longer and less damaged the protective tips, the less likely the shoelaces are to become damaged themselves. Telomere length is a predictor of overall mortality.[45]

Exposure to environmental stressors such as pollution, smoking, poor diet and alcohol, as well as chronic stress and poor sleep quality, are associated with telomere shortening. Changes at the cellular level are associated with premature ageing and premature death from diseases such as cancer and heart disease. You can now send off for tests which claim to provide you with your biological age by measuring telomere length from a drop of blood, but such tests have been criticised for being unreliable, as well as the fact that it isn't clear what the information means for an individual's health.[46] There are also various online tools, which, by asking you a series of lifestyle questions, purport to give you your 'true body age'.

Some scientists argue that biological or cellular ageing is the most significant risk factor for almost all diseases and there is increasing interest in scientific studies that suggest the effects of ageing (or senescence) are reversible through therapeutic interventions. Jim Mellon and Al Chalabi, entrepreneurs with an interest in investment, have written about developments in biological and molecular science in their book *Juvenescence*. They see huge opportunities for investors in the longevity market, which is developing and commercialising products that will reverse the effects of ageing.

So it's no surprise that large bio-tech companies have made multi-billion-dollar investments into researching and developing therapeutic innovations designed to 'cure' ageing. By targeting the underlying ageing process, rather than just one disease, these new treatments hold out the promise of extending the years we spend in good health and could revolutionise the treatment of diseases and challenge much current medical practice, medical research and drug treatments.

The World Health Organisation produces an International Classification of Diseases which is the 'bible' for doctors and health services worldwide. What's recorded officially in here gets reimbursed. In a lot of countries, the way that hospitals and other health services are paid, both by private insurers as well as social insurance and government-funded care, is based on this classification. Regulations of drugs and devices which assess whether treatments are safe and the price that will be paid also reference this 'bible', so it's a big deal that in its 2018 update the World Health Organisation included for the first time a code for 'old age'.[47] The inclusion of 'old age' as a disease or condition means it can *legitimately be treated by doctors*. This opens the door for drug therapies designed to slow the process of ageing to be used in clinical care, potentially worth billions of dollars to these companies.

Currently, you go and see an oncologist if you have cancer, a neurologist if you have Parkinson's Disease or a rheumatologist if you have rheumatoid arthritis. In future you might just need to see a geriatrician, but instead of offering 'care for the elderly' they might be offering a 'cure for ageing'. But at what cost?

If it can be monetised by the drug companies, there is a risk that ageing becomes heavily medicalised, but Zoe Wyrko argues for the opposite aim: 'We need to de-medicalise everything. We need to start looking at the whole life course. While doctors and GPs and hospitals are really important, there is *so much more* that is people's own responsibility rather than my health being seen as somebody else's problem.' Doctors reinforce this with their paternalism, she argues. We might also need to change our attitudes, not expecting to come away from the doctors with a prescription for a drug, but welcoming advice or a prescription for exercise or diet.

Science is giving us new insights into the biological processes of ageing and these developments are attracting lots of investment from industry in the hope of finding a 'cure' for ageing. Yet we risk worsening inequalities if only those who can afford them get access or bankrupting the NHS due to the likely cost of these novel treatments.

We have a choice between a medicalised and bio-pharma industrialised response to ageing, which sees it as yet another thing that doctors can treat, or we can embrace the opportunity of longevity and focus on maximising the years spent in good health through the things we already know work. Far from making the case for more widespread testing and treatment of 'ageing', these insights further underline that the key to healthy ageing lies in reducing the lifetime of exposure to risk factors, such as smoking and alcohol. It gives even greater weight to why we need to invest in prevention.

There are those who blame older people for the woes of the NHS. Yet the biggest driver of spending is the intensity of treatment, particularly in the last two years of life. Medicalising old age and spending huge sums of money to delay the inevitable – death – won't give us the happy and healthy later life we all wish for, either. We need a radical rethink of our attitude to death and whether we should keep people alive at all costs.

Nor are health services about to be overwhelmed by a tidal wave of sick old people. The problem is that the current model of health care is broken. It sees older people as a collection of diseases and fails to provide the support and proactive care needed earlier to help people with chronic conditions live as well as possible. And when people with chronic conditions do need acute care, this needs to be delivered in an integrated way that recognises the complexities of multi-morbidity.

Despite the hype surrounding scientific breakthroughs that could 'cure' ageing, they distract from the simpler steps we could take to prevent the causes of premature ageing. This will require a serious focus on prevention and reducing inequalities. Targeted action to change people's behaviours will not be enough. It requires bold action by government. Action needs to be taken to address the life-long causes of ill health, such as smoking, alcohol consumption and obesity, to give future generations the best chance of a healthy old age.

However successful we are at keeping ourselves healthy for as long as possible, many of us will suffer the effects of disease or disability or experience some loss of ability due to wear and tear towards the end of our lives. This can impact our ability to remain independent. Many of us will need some help with everyday living. In the next chapter I look at the impact of the age shift on social care.

7

Who cares?

'It's time to declare a social care emergency.'
Anonymous social worker, *The Guardian* (August 2019)[1]

As well as pressures on the NHS, we're also worried sick as a nation about who will look after us if we're frail. TV programmes investigate abuse and mistreatment in care homes, cementing a view that moving to one is to be avoided at all costs. Many of us will also have experienced caring for an older relative, struggling to access the care and support they need, shocked at the costs and perhaps making the difficult decision to move them to a care home, only to find a limited number of suitable places available, and a complex system of assessments and entitlements. So how will we care for the growing number of older people with long-term care needs? Are there alternatives to the care home we should be investing in now?

The lack of adequate funding for social care means that the burden of care increasingly falls on unpaid family carers. But can these carers fill the gap left by the cuts in local authority care? With people having fewer children (or no children), there is a risk that there will be no-one to care for us when we get old. How are changing patterns of households, families and work going to impact on the supply of informal care?

Old age is associated with decline and frailty, problems we mostly don't want to talk about and certainly don't want to imagine ourselves with, like memory loss, incontinence or losing our sight. Does old age mean an inevitable loss of fitness and independence? Or are there things we can do to prevent us getting frail? Having considered the implications of the age shift for the NHS in the last chapter, here I look in more detail at the impact on social care.

WHAT IS THE CURRENT STATE OF SOCIAL CARE?

We hear frequently on the news that care homes are shutting down and many others are on the brink of bankruptcy. We also hear heart-rending stories of relatives or friends overburdened by having to care for elderly relatives who are not eligible for funding from the local council for home care support or for a place in a care home. People who do go into a care home pay a fortune in fees and their homes have to be sold to pay for care when the cash runs out. Social care is about to collapse and needs a massive injection of funding. How true is this gloomy picture? There are certainly widespread problems with the current system of care and the support available to older people with care needs, as you will know if you have tried to access care and support for a relative or partner.

There are challenges with recruiting and retaining staff, particularly nurses. Skills for Care, the strategic independent body for workforce development in adult social care, estimated there were over 100,000 vacancies in adult social care in 2018.[2] Demand for formal carers is also projected to increase, with one 2014 projection suggesting that 1 million additional carers would be needed by 2025.[3]

Local authority funding cuts have meant that care is provided to fewer people and in many places only to those with the highest levels of need. Between 2009-2010 and 2016-2017 some estimated 400,000 people have not received care who would previously have been eligible, as resources have been focused on those people with the highest and most critical levels of need.[4] The financial threshold at which the means test applies has also not risen with inflation since 2010-2011, which means people with savings and assets of more than £23,250 are not eligible for local authority-funded care. There is therefore a significant unmet need, leaving family carers, the voluntary and charity sector and individuals to provide lower levels of care and support in people's homes and in the community.

The Local Government Association estimates that adult social care services in England face a funding gap of £3.5 billion by 2025.[5] The Care Quality Commission, the independent regulator of health and social care services in England, has also recently issued warnings about the financial position of some care home providers, including Allied Health, which operates across 84 councils in England. When Southern Cross (one of the biggest care home operators in England) went bust in 2011, councils were required to find alternative places for some 30,000 residents while administrators sought to secure buyers who would continue to operate the homes. As a result, the Care Quality Commission was required by the Government to monitor the financial position of the largest operators and to provide early warnings of insolvencies. There are still problems, though, as the market is highly fragmented, and characterised by a few large operators and many small independent businesses. The combination of the reduction in the amount local authorities pay to providers of care, increases in the minimum wage, and the quality and safety requirements of regulators have pushed many care homes into debt. At time of writing in 2019, the latest high-profile company to go into administration was Four Seasons Healthcare, which had 17,000 residents across 322 care homes.

There are broadly two types of care home: nursing homes and residential homes. Residential homes are not able to take people who need medical or nursing care. These homes are suitable for those people who need assistance with daily living, such as bathing and dressing, and provide a secure place to live with company and social activities. The level of need of people in care homes is changing. More care home residents have dementia or are close to end of life. There has therefore been a significant increase in the number of nursing home beds compared to residential home beds.[6] There are much higher levels of dependency among care home residents today, people who would have been in hospices or long-stay old-age hospital wards in the past.[7] Fewer people with lower level needs are receiving any care and even those with moderate needs have to stay in their own homes with some home care support.

Even with this growth in demand for home care services, there are problems. A recent assessment of home care services in England by leading health think-tank, The King's Fund, concluded that, 'The future of home care is uncertain, and the market is fragile ... Home care agencies struggle to recruit and retain staff. Quality is far from uniform.'[8] Home care providers reported significant difficulties recruiting in more affluent areas, where wages are generally higher and fewer people are willing to work on zero-hour contracts or in low-paying jobs, and in rural areas, where workers are reluctant to travel the long distances between clients. As many as 41% of care providers were found by Her Majesty's Revenue and Customs to be paying below the minimum wage because they were not paying travel time.[9] A court case in 2013 ruled that time between visits should be paid unless the worker had sufficient time to return home between appointments. Low pay was also highlighted as an issue by providers, who criticised local authority commissioning models that awarded contracts to the lowest bidder. Some of these providers could not fulfil their contract and services had to be picked up by other providers. Despite increasing demand, there has been long-term pay stagnation for most staff in the care sector because of the low fees paid by local authorities to providers and the increased costs of providing care.[10]

Unless there is a dramatic increase in the amount that local authorities pay to care home providers and home care companies (which is only possible if the Government increases funding to local authorities or Council Tax and business rates increase significantly), it is likely this trend will continue. Many homes have managed to stay afloat by cross-subsidising the fees paid by private clients, but increasingly homes are simply refusing to

THE AGE OF AGEING BETTER?

admit local authority-funded residents or require their families to top up the fees, sometimes asking them to pay significant amounts. The average fee in England for a place in a residential home is £2,691 a month. That rises to £3,796 per month for a place in a nursing home, where the person has higher levels of medical need.[11] Eligibility for social care funding varies across the countries of the UK. However, in general, for those with very few savings and assets, the local authority will pay the cost of a basic care home place. For those with some assets, they only get partial support and will have to contribute to the costs of care (except in Wales where people are either eligible for support or are self-funders). In total, service users in England contributed £2.7 billion in care costs for adults in 2017-2018.[12]

Despite these financial pressures, service standards do continue to improve. The Care Quality Commission inspects all providers of adult social care. In its annual report on *The State of Health Care and Adult Social Care in England in 2017/18*, it highlighted that the number of providers rated outstanding has increased and, of those that were rated inadequate, nearly 90% have improved their rating.[13] So despite the headlines, and in the face of real and severe challenges, the majority of providers are providing safe care and quality is improving.

The provision of formal care services, though, is clearly quite precarious, whether we are talking about residential and nursing home providers or home care providers. Cuts in local authority funding have not only pushed providers to the edge financially, but mean they are cut to the bone in terms of providing a quality service. The reduction in eligibility to only those with the highest levels of need (and without income or assets) has shifted responsibility for care, both providing it and funding it, onto family members. Can families fill the gap?

CAN UNPAID FAMILY CARE FILL THE GAP?

At the last census, in 2011, nearly 20% of people over 50 reported providing unpaid care, with 26% of these providing more than

50 hours of care a week.[14] But families are shrinking, with people having fewer children and a significant minority having no children, restricting the pool of potential family carers. Even for those with children, those children may not be willing to provide that level of personal care. The propensity of family members to become carers is influenced by their own financial situation, health and geographic proximity. Women who have traditionally been relied on to provide the lion's share of care, either for their spouse or partner or for a parent or relative, are now more likely to be juggling a job as well. There is projected to be a significant decline in the availability of informal care, with smaller families, more people ageing without children and more people working later in life, as well as changing expectations and attitudes, both of older adults who don't want to be cared for by family members and the lack of willingness of relatives to provide personal care.[15] Other trends, such as men and women now living to similar ages, rising divorce rates and the rise in people living alone, and for some groups, family members living far apart, all have an impact on the availability of informal or unpaid family care.

Research that tries to predict the demand for informal care and the likely supply of care givers in the light of these social and demographic changes shows there is already a 'care gap' which will only widen in future. Within five years, there is projected to be a shortfall of nearly a million informal carers, rising to 2.3 million in 2035.[16] Overall, it is pretty clear that if family members are not able to fill the care gap it will mean more demand on already stretched local authority social care services or families having to pay for private care themselves.

My brother-in-law is in his mid-40s and is not working in order to provide care for my mother-in-law. As a result, there has been very little cost to social care. Other than someone to bathe her on discharge from hospital following surgery for cancer and to change dressings for a very brief time, my brother-in-law has provided the bulk of the care. But being a full-time carer has an impact on his life and his ability to work, and therefore his financial position, both now and later in life.

His situation underlines the need for employers to support working carers, as we saw in chapter 4, but there is a need for more universal support for all carers. We need proper financial support for carers. Since 2010 carers do at least get credits for National Insurance so their entitlement to a state pension is not negatively affected by not being in work. However, the level of benefit received as a carer is only £64.60 per week from Carer's Allowance, compared to £73.10 for both Income Support and Job Seeker's Allowance. Eligibility is based on whether the person you're caring for is in receipt of Attendance Allowance (the main disability benefit for people over the state pension age) or other disability benefits (for those below state pension age). Even if the carer claims Income Support and the Carer's Premium they have less than £9,000 to live off a year. As a society, if we value caring and recognise the increased costs to health and social care if it were not there, informal carers need to be properly valued through the benefits system, by increasing Carer's Allowance to at least match Jobseeker's Allowance.

Currently in the UK, eligibility for local authority-funded care takes into account the availability of informal care. In other words, if there is someone who can care for you, your needs are deemed to be lower than someone who is on their own and as a result you may get less support (if any). Other countries have more universal systems of long-term care which are carer 'blind'. In other words, eligibility is primarily based on disability. For example, in Germany the assessment is based on need and the funding you are eligible for can be used to pay a family carer or for professional carers. In Japan, where the assessment is also based on need, funding must be used to pay for professional carers not family members. This was done because they wanted to encourage people, particularly women, to remain active in work rather than take on family caring responsibilities. As we saw on page 87 in chapter 4, there is a shortage of care workers in Japan to provide this formal care.

Either more needs to be done to encourage and support people to provide family care or else there will need to be a lot more spent, both privately and by the state, on formal care services. Unless there is urgent reform to the funding and provision of social care in the UK, more people will be spending more of their later life providing unpaid care to older parents or to spouses or to both. While this caregiving is hugely valuable, it can have a detrimental impact on the care giver. It reinforces gender inequalities as the burden of care falls particularly on women (they are twice as likely to be carers under the age of 65 than men). It can also result in early exit from the labour market, and carers are at higher risk of social isolation and loneliness, making it harder for them to sustain their social networks.[17]

Relying on informal care is unlikely to meet growing demand and has significant consequences for those who provide unpaid care. As we've seen in chapter 5, people in later life increasingly spend a lot of their time providing care for loved ones, but it is vital that as a society we increase the amount of public spending on social care to guarantee everyone the dignity of having care and support to remain as independent as possible in old age.

WHAT ARE WE WILLING TO PAY?

The fact is that we need to spend more on social care than we do. The UK urgently needs a long-term political consensus on social care funding, recognising the need for increased public funding and not just putting the financial burden on those who use care. We need to share the risk. It shouldn't matter if someone has long-term care needs or dies of a short illness, the state, and therefore everyone through taxation, should support them equally. It is this desire for fairness that was at the heart of opposition to the social care proposals in the Conservative Party's manifesto for the 2017 general election.

Most people don't realise that the value of their home is at risk to pay for social care. Currently only £14,250 is protected. The proposal was to increase the protected amount. For those with property, this was an improvement on the current system, but because the majority of the public were not aware that any of the value of their property could be used to pay for social care, there was a very strong and negative backlash. The proposal was dubbed the 'dementia tax'. People felt it was deeply unfair to have most illnesses cared for free at the point of need by the NHS, but others – like dementia – subject to higher payments by individuals, because dementia care is largely provided in non-NHS settings. The criticism caused Prime Minister Theresa May to have to withdraw the proposal.

LONG-TERM CARE INSURANCE IN GERMANY

Since 1995, long-term care insurance (LTCI) has been compulsory in Germany. For people in work, the cost of this is split equally between employee and employer. It is the role of the Federal Employment Agency to make both contributions on behalf of people out of work, but how LTCI funds work varies from one federal state to another. This insurance sits alongside four other mandatory insurance schemes for employers (health, unemployment, pension and accident insurance). Most health care insurance funds, which are mostly run at a regional level, also have a LTCI component. This does not cover everything; for example, the 'hotel' cost of residential care is excluded and must be paid by the resident themselves. After retirement the person must pay the full contribution themselves. Around 90% of the population is covered by state LTCI and most of the remaining 10%, for example, freelancers or high-earners, can choose to purchase private LTCI.

To access the scheme, an assessment is carried out and service users are categorised according to five levels of need, with one being the highest level of need. To qualify, people need to have at least two years' worth of contributions, but since this is not 'old-age care insurance', there is no age requirement. Reforms in 2015-2017 also added a 'level zero' for those diagnosed with dementia and those with cognitive difficulties but not yet requiring high levels of personal care.

The benefit applies to both home-based and residential care. There is a large degree of flexibility for those accessing home-based care. They can generally choose between cash benefits for informal care givers and benefits in kind, i.e. services like domiciliary care or cash payments towards residential care. Of the 3.4 million beneficiaries of LTCI in 2017, 80% chose cash benefits. LTCI benefits vary, but many provide support such as training in basic nursing skills and respite care for informal carers, as well as money to make low-cost changes to the home, such as specialist furniture or to improve accessibility.[18]

The system is entirely self-funding and contributions are capped at about 2.5% a month, adjusted for income. For those over the age of 23, there is an additional 0.25% surcharge for those who do not have children, as it is assumed that those with children will receive some care free of charge from them. In Germany, 21% of women born in 1967 did not have children by 2017, when they turned 50.[19] This is only slightly higher than the 19% of British women born in 1967 who did not have children by the time they are 45.[20]

The introduction of LTCI meant a rapid reduction in the amount that federal states had to pay in social security benefits to those who could not afford care, and evaluations of LTCI have suggested an increased sense of security, especially for those on middle incomes, and an increase in the number of people able to receive care in their homes, as well as a concurrent reduction in those over 65 living with their children.[21]

Both Germany and Japan have introduced compulsory social insurance to fund long-term care (see box above), but a National Insurance levy is not necessarily a good idea. It restricts the tax base to those in employment and National Insurance is currently not paid by those working after state pension age. We have to look at a wider tax base which would involve taxing things other than earnings – such as capital, wealth or inheritance. Given the large accumulation of wealth among older generations through house price rises and revaluation of the defined benefit pension schemes, it seems fair to look at how these assets can be taxed, by, for example, increasing inheritance tax or taxes on pension income.

Fixing social care also means addressing the eligibility for NHS Continuing Care, which enables people with a medical condition but who require some long-term care to apply for this to be funded by the NHS. Given the high costs of social care, particularly to individuals and families who are not eligible for means-tested funding from their local authority, passing this assessment makes a huge difference.

The NHS Continuing Care process came about following the court case of Pamela Coughlan in 1999. Although Coughlan is tetraplegic, at the time she did not have significant additional health needs, so her local NHS tried to transfer responsibility for her care to the local authority. However, the judge ruled that Coughlan's health needs were above the level the local authority could or should provide and so the NHS had an ongoing obligation to continue to pay for her care. A National Framework for NHS Continuing Care was subsequently released to ensure local authority policies were in line with the principles established in the Coughlan case. In 2015-2016, almost 160,000 people received, or were assessed as eligible for, NHS Continuing Care funding. NHS England estimates that spending on Continuing Health Care, NHS-funded nursing care and assessment costs will increase from £3,607 million in 2015-2016 to £5,247 million in 2020-2021.[22] The eligibility for NHS Continuing Care reinforces the differences between those who get free or subsidised care, such as someone with cancer, and those who don't, such as someone with dementia, because their medical needs are not significant enough.

Instead of raising more funds we *could* radically redistribute the money currently spent on the NHS. The Better Care Fund,

a step towards integration of health and social care by pooling
funds between the two services, did not go far enough and did not
clearly remove the differences between health care – a national
service that is universal and (largely) free at the point of use –
on the one hand, and social care – locally funded heavily means
tested, with user charges – on the other. Labour advocated
for a National Care Service in order to remove this division
when Andy Burnham, now Mayor of Greater Manchester, was
Secretary of State for Health in 2010. The proposal was to
make social care universal and fund it from general taxation. In
other words, it would no longer be means tested and, although
money would be collected centrally, it was still to pass to local
authorities to commission and deliver services. While eligibility
was to be set nationally, the proposal was not for all social care
to be free at the point of use like the NHS, but rather to protect
people from catastrophic costs, such as more than two years
in a care home. The initial steps were limited to extending free
personal care for people being cared for in their own home to
England (a policy that was already in operation in Scotland).
This was never implemented and subsequent governments have
failed to address the fundamental unfairness between the NHS
and social care.

The current system, which rests on defining what is health
care and what is social care, what is nursing care versus personal
care, who is eligible for NHS Continuing Care and who isn't,
what different levels of need for care people have and how many
assets people have, leaves families bewildered and professionals
unable to deliver high-quality care in the most suitable setting
for an individual. While a single national health and care service,
funded by taxation and free at the point of need is highly
improbable, a rethink is needed to address the fundamental
fault lines that run between health and social care. One option
might be to distinguish between (short-term) acute medical care
and (long-term) nursing and social care, similar to the system
of public long-term care insurance in the Netherlands, which
was in place until 2015. While coverage of this was generous,

including residential care, home care, community nursing and social assistance for the elderly, it was judged to be inefficient and created incentives to admit people to institutional settings. Reforms in the Netherlands mean that the long-term care insurance since 2015 only provides care to those who need it 24/7. Lower-level needs are now met through a social assistance programme provided by the municipalities. As in the UK, local budgets have been cut and there is therefore a higher reliance on families and informal community support.[23]

The pressures on social care are real and urgent. We cannot get away from the need to properly fund social care. This is vital if care providers are to attract, train and reward the workforce, to ensure standards are met and deliver quality care. This raises difficult questions about what we are collectively willing to pay for, or whether we will accept limits on the care available or indeed the quality of care. We need to balance this with a call to action to do more to prevent the *need* for social care by promoting healthy ageing and reducing dependency.

In a moment I'll look at some of the potential ways in which care provided to older people in future will change, but first let's consider how the levels of need are changing and whether the decline in our abilities is inevitable.

HOW MUCH CARE WILL WE NEED?

For most us independence at a most basic level means being able to look after ourselves without help from someone else, particularly for activities such as bathing, dressing, making meals and going to the shops. When we are no longer able to carry out these everyday activities, called activities of daily living, we need care and support. This is one way in which we are considered to be 'disabled' or 'dependent'. So how many of us can expect to become dependent and for how long?

There is mixed evidence on whether the rates of disability at older ages, as measured by daily living activities, are rising or falling. According to the 2017 Health Survey for England, prevalence of disability among older adults is falling. The percentage of over-65s needing help with at least one activity of daily living fell from 32% in 2011 to 26% in 2017.[24] The Family Resources Survey, a larger survey of 19,000 households, found a higher level of disability with 45% of pension-age adults reporting they had substantial difficulties with activities of daily living.[25]

The Cognitive Function and Ageing Studies (CFAS) are detailed studies of levels of dependency (including the intensity and frequency of help required), led by researchers at Newcastle University. In 2017 they found there had been an 'expansion of dependency'. Life expectancy for men and women at age 65 years rose between 1991 and 2011, but these extra years have been lived with care needs – an additional 2.4 years for men and for women an additional 3 years with some level of dependency.[26] If these trends continue it means there will be many more people living with care needs for longer. While the researchers noted that fewer older people with substantial care needs now reside in care homes, if the current pattern of care home usage remained the same, they estimated an extra 71,215 care home places will be needed by 2025.

The same CFAS study also looked at the amount of time on average we spend at different levels of dependency. The three levels of dependency were: low dependency, defined as needing help less than once a day with tasks such as shopping or housework; medium, requiring help several times a day, for example, with dressing and preparing meals; and high, requiring care 24 hours a day, usually because of an inability to go to the toilet or feed themselves unaided, severe cognitive impairment or limited mobility. Researchers found that on average a man aged 65 years old now could expect to live 17.6 years, of which he could expect to be fully independent with no care needs for 11.2 years, a further 4 years with low dependency, just over a year with moderate dependency and 1.3 years with the highest level of dependency.

As there is with life expectancy, there are inequalities in disability. The number of years lived with a disability is considerably higher

ABOUT THE FRAILTY INDEX

The Electronic Frailty Index, developed in 2018 by a team including Martin Vernon, a leading geriatrician and former National Clinical Director for Older People at NHS England, is now being adopted by GP practices. The index can be used to categorise patients into one of several groups – fit (meaning not frail), mild, moderate or severe frailty – based on a number of different measures, including diagnosis of a range of chronic diseases, physical impairments such as reduced hearing or sight, other symptoms like urinary incontinence or memory problems, and some more social ones such as whether the person is housebound. The idea behind this is to be able to plan and design services based on the numbers of people in each category. At an individual level it can be used to target services better, according to someone's level of frailty rather than assumptions based on age. For example, for those with mild or moderate frailty, the aim should be to maintain their ability to function and, where possible, reverse the decline through rehabilitation, i.e. strength and balance classes. Those with severe frailty may need more intense care and support with a focus on preventing a fall or undernutrition.

Preventing people from becoming frail has significant cost implications for the NHS and social care, with the average cost of a person with severe frailty being approximately £7,000 – twice as much as the cost of someone who has mild frailty and nearly six times the cost of someone who is fit.[27] It is the higher cost of community and social care that accounts for the difference rather than the cost of acute hospital care or GP visits, because people with severe frailty need help with day-to-day care rather than more medical treatment.

in deprived areas than it is in wealthier areas. In 2015-2017, a baby boy born in Blackpool had a disability-free life expectancy of 54.8 years, compared to 71.2 in Sutton – a disability-free life expectancy gap of more than 16 years.[28]

Doctors in the UK have recently developed a new way of measuring how frail or how fit people over 65 are, called the Electronic Frailty Index (see box on page 188). According to analysis of data from the population in Kent, 45% of people over 70 are fit and as many as one in five over 90 are also fit. It is important not to assume that just because of someone's age they will be frail and need help. The vast majority of people who are frail are in their 80s and 90s. One in 10 over-85s experience severe frailty compared to just two in a 100 in their 70s. This reinforces the need to focus on maintaining fitness and health among people in their 60s and 70s, and underlines that someone shouldn't be labelled as 'frail' just because they're old, which is something that geriatrician Dr Zoe Wyrko warns against. She says that while frailty is important as a medical term, it needs to be used appropriately following a clinical assessment. She says it shouldn't be used by doctors 'just because I've seen them in a hospital bed and they're skinny and their hair's a mess because they've had pneumonia and they're wearing a horrible hospital nightie, and nobody's bothered to clean their teeth for three days.'

As well as preventing ill-health, though, are there things we can do to reduce disability and dependency, which are key factors in the demand for social care?

REDUCING DEPENDENCY AT OLDER AGES

Whether we are physically active can make a huge difference not only to our health, but also to whether we can carry out everyday activities and it plays a significant role in preventing falls. Around a third of people 65 and over fall at least once a year,[29] but we can do something about this by tackling an aspect of physical activity that is particularly important as we get older – strengthening our muscles and improving our balance.

There is strong evidence that strength and balance exercises can reverse muscle wasting and thereby prevent falls.[30] From the age of 40 we lose 8% of muscle mass a decade, rising to 15% once we reach 70.[31] Falls are the most common reason for death by injury for people over 65 and cost the NHS on average £2,600 to treat. Falls can also result in hip fractures, after which one in three people die within a year.[32] If we lose our muscle strength, it can impact our 'get up and go' time; that is the time it takes us to stand up from a chair, walk three metres, walk back and sit down. This can make the difference between making it to the toilet unaided or not. If we lose the ability to get to the loo, this is the difference between needing a care package where someone pops in twice a day to your home to help with washing and dressing, and needing 24/7 care, associated with a five-fold difference in costs.[33]

A review of evidence, published by Public Health England and overseen by the UK Chief Medical Officers' Expert Committee for muscle strength, bone health and balance, recommended exercise at least twice a week which includes high intensity resistance training, some impact training such as running, and balance training.[34] There is some evidence that everyday activities such as gardening and carrying shopping can help improve muscle strength, but the evidence supports resistance and circuit training, and ball and racquet sports as having the strongest effect on muscle and bone strength and balance. Some types of dance and movement, such as Tai Chi, are also beneficial, though the strength of the effect is lower.[35] The Royal Academy of Dance runs ballet classes across the country designed for people over 55 called Silver Swans. Their oldest dancer is 102! There are well-evidenced physical and mental benefits to dance classes, aside from enjoyment itself. Ballet, especially, can improve mobility, strength and balance, which can in turn protect against falls and ill health generally. And for those who don't fancy ballet or tea dances, there is always Zumba Gold – classes that are designed for the 'young at heart'!

The same review found that for older adults who are at high risk of falling a more structured and targeted programme of exercise, which includes resistance training, is beneficial. While some local areas commission these structured and evidence-based programmes, availability is patchy, they don't always target those who can benefit, and they often don't support people to sustain the activities after the end of the programme.[36] Aesop, a social enterprise and charity, has developed an evidence-based community dance programme called Dance to Health, which is designed to reduce falls. It's a national programme, popular with men as well as women (who are more at risk of falls because of osteoporosis). Participation rates tend to remain high in these programmes, because they are creative, fun and sociable.

People who are sedentary are at higher risk of falling, as are people who are admitted to hospital or a care home, as they are more likely to be sitting down or in bed for long periods of time and this can lead to a (further) loss of mobility, strength and balance. People need to be helped to get up and be mobile, both during hospital stays and after they are discharged. Oomph is a national initiative that delivers group-based exercises, mainly to care homes (see box below).

CHAIR-BASED EXERCISES WITH OOMPH

The classes are inclusive and usually chair-based, such as chair aerobics or chair cheerleading. In 2017-2018, Oomph delivered 45,400 exercise classes in care homes and trained 322 instructors in the community. Client feedback has been hugely positive, with 98% saying that the classes had a beneficial impact on their residents. Wholesale evaluation of the scheme is in its early stages, but there are indications that the programme has helped to reduce falls and increase physical mobility in many of the care homes it does classes in.[37]

Activity – physical, cognitive and emotional – is key to keeping older people fitter and healthier for longer. Professor Sir Muir Gray, a long-time advocate of physical activity argues, 'If we started training people in their 80s and 90s now, then we could probably make an impact as soon as the following winter. In three months, you can strengthen the core reserves of people in their 90s.' He goes on to explain that if people have diminished reserves – when they get an infection, for example – it aggravates any underlying conditions, such as heart failure or respiratory problems. The body's response means that the person can't get out of their chair. Doctors refer to them as 'off their legs'. Muir is adamant that we need to challenge the orthodoxy that 'rest is best' and that people should take it easy. His solution: 'a bonfire of the slippers'.

Dr Zoe Wyrko, who assessed residents in the care home that hosted a nursery in the Channel 4 show *Old People's Home for 4 Year Olds*, is convinced it's possible to reverse some of the loss of function we see in older people. She puts many of the improvements in both physical and cognitive function that were seen in the older residents on the TV show down to improvements in confidence. 'I think for most of the older people featured on the programme, most of the physical improvements were down to psychological improvements. We did no specific exercises with them to improve strength really, nothing specific to improve brain power, just doing standard activities that are normal things to do with children. We saw confidence going up and it's having that confidence in your own abilities that is the biggest thing we can do to help people view ageing differently. Really educating people that bodies and brains change as you age, but the impact need not be quite as big as we make it out to be. And, yes, there are things that need to be made easier, but you can make things easier for someone without taking away their independence.'

Zoe thinks that sometimes family members, carers and health professionals do too much for older people, de-skilling them, reducing their confidence, when in fact they are still capable of doing these things for themselves, particularly if the environment is adapted to make things easier (this is something I'll come onto in chapter 8). She told me about Sylvia aged 103 who was on the programme (see box opposite).

SYLVIA'S STORY

Sylvia, aged 103, is a resident of Lark Hill Retirement Village. She was wrapped in cotton wool by her family, allowed to walk around her room, but otherwise put in a wheelchair to be wheeled about. She came in with a diagnosis of mild cognitive impairment and possible early dementia. If she didn't know the answer to the question, she would giggle or make a rude joke. At the start of the programme, if you'd said, 'Sylvia, did you bring a coat?', she'd just giggle at you and say, 'What do you think, dear?', as in 'I really can't remember.' She did appear typical of someone with cognitive impairment who will sit in a room with activities going on around them and are happy to be there, but are not interacting at all until somebody comes over and talks to them.

It was about six weeks in when goats had been brought in to encourage movement. Sylvia absolutely loved the goats. I think she'd had them as a child, so was familiar with them. Everyone else had gone out to lunch, but then Sylvia turned around and walked back into the room. We thought she had come back for a sneaky pat of the goats while the kids were all gone, but she picked her handbag up off the back of the chair and walked out. The fact that she was able to remember that she'd brought a handbag with her, and to go back and get it, was amazing.

There is now more independence, because her family can see that she can do more than they had allowed her to do. At the end of the programme, they told Zoe they'd noticed how much more awake and alert she was, and that she'd been telling them stories about her youth that they'd never heard before. They'd seen her becoming different. Put Sylvia in a room now and she'll be looking at what's going on and who she can interact with, and she didn't do that at the start.

Getting everyone moving at older ages and ensuring active rehabilitation to restore people's function, following, for example, a hospital stay, could make a big difference to the demand for social care. But given the large increase in the population aged over 85 over the next decade or more, even if we do achieve huge improvements in people's muscle strength and balance, there will still be a need to care for people. If we are to provide high-quality care and support for everyone in future, there needs to be a revolution in care-giving.

A REVOLUTION IN CARE-GIVING

Cuts in local government budgets mean that care services have been stripped back to the bare minimum. Most care staff receive little training and are paid the minimum wage. A 15-minute visit is the norm, leaving the carer little time to get someone up, washed, dressed and fed, never mind develop a relationship with the person, but some providers in the private sector are bucking the trend. For example, Home Instead specifically recruits carers on the basis that they have the values and attitudes to build a caring relationship with the person – and there are plenty of other innovative models being tried out. They are more expensive and it can still be a challenge in rural areas to get home care services, even if you are willing to pay.

Ideas abound about how to meet growing demand for care and some hold out the promise that technology will revolutionise how care is delivered. At the moment technology is used to monitor residents in care homes, for example, with sensors on mattresses so care staff are alerted if someone tries to get out of bed unaided or two-way video links between care home residents and doctors in a clinical hub.[38] Similar technology can be fitted in people's homes so relatives are alerted if their loved ones don't get out of bed or open their fridge at particular times. Products like Canary Care allow you to remotely monitor movement, temperature and blood pressure. It is a sensor system, rather than a surveillance system, and doesn't use cameras or microphones.

Other technologies include beds that can detect seizures and alert carers, and a pre-programmed watch that reminds people to take their medication.

Adaptations and technology can help with cognitive decline and dementia, too. For example, guardian angel/dementia buddy devices can allow people to assist someone with dementia who is living at home. These devices are commonly worn as a wristband, badge, bag tag or keyring and work in a similar way to contactless bank cards. If a person can't remember how to get home or is distressed and has a 'tap here' tag, tapping it with a mobile phone will give you their address and a number to contact in an emergency. Technology can also help those with sensory impairment, such as a talking hob that automatically switches off when the timer goes off. The latest buzz is about smart homes fitted with devices and appliances that can be monitored or accessed remotely, via a smartphone or computer, to control temperature, lights, or indeed any aspect of the home environment.

Accelerometers in smartphones can already detect if someone has had a fall and automatically alert guardians. In the future data from wearable devices on walking speed and gait may also be able to sense changes in movement associated with the early signs of dementia or could predict whether someone is likely to have a fall. While these gadgets could be reassuring for family members, as yet there is little evidence that they reduce falls or improve outcomes for people. However, a government-funded evaluation of telehealth interventions (that combines clinical advice, classes about your condition and group interaction with other patients via your TV), called the Whole System Demonstrator Programme, found some tentative evidence that telehealth can reduce mortality, the need for admissions to hospital, the number of bed days in hospital and the time spent in A&E.[39]

Surveillance of this sort has raised ethical questions about the intrusion on privacy and the level of control that is appropriate. While it may give peace of mind to family members or enable carers to check on patients without actually seeing them, it will inevitably reduce human contact, reducing the physiological benefits of touch, as well as reducing social contact for those who are housebound, for example.

Robotics is another area where there is much hype about the opportunities to transform the care of people with dementia, mobility issues and other care needs. Robots like Paro the robotic seal are being used in the care of people with dementia as 'therapy pets' that like being stroked and held. Early findings from a review of research studies of these technologies showed that they are being used in a range of ways and some studies have shown they are associated with positive outcomes on mood, reduced agitation, depression and loneliness, and increased sociability. However, some studies found that the effects of the robotic seal were no different from those of a soft toy or switched-off robot, and a robotic pet seems to produce similar effects in providing companionship as a real pet.[40] So while there is potential to use technology to enhance care, we need to design it with the users in mind, test the benefits and minimise the undesirable consequences, like reduced social interaction or touch from real humans!

Some of the robotic innovations being developed by labs in two universities in Bristol are designed to assist people with tasks in the home to enable independent living. One robot that I saw demonstrated worked a bit like a self-operating hoist and was helping someone with limited mobility to get up from their seat or bed and walk across the room. Devices like this could free up care workers from heavy manual lifting, so that they can focus more on the psychological, social and emotional aspects of care.

While care homes are on the brink of bankruptcy it seems very unlikely that there will be a major investment in innovation and adoption of these technologies any time soon. Even if they substitute for staff, given most care workers are on the minimum wage, it is not clear that technological substitutes will be cheaper. And as we will see in chapter 8, for individuals living in damp, cold, hazardous homes, perhaps unable to access the toilet or bath unaided, other much more basic improvements and adaptations are needed before starting to invest in technology.

There are other innovations and models of care that are not technology-led but offer different ways of providing care and support outside a care home setting. Here are a few examples:

- SharedLives plus runs a Homeshare scheme that enables older people with low level needs to rent a room to a young person. There are mutual benefits for both the homeowner and homesharer, with the older person perhaps getting help with keeping on top of housework and the younger person paying reduced rent in return for these tasks. While this is quite common in other countries like France, it has not yet taken off across the UK.
- Carerooms is like an Airbnb for people who need a place to rest and recover, perhaps on discharge from hospital before going home. The organisation carefully vets hosts and inspects the rooms to make sure they are suitable and safe for the person.
- Supercarers is an online platform that connects people with experienced carers in their area, cutting out the agency and allowing a direct relationship between the family and the carer. A range of services are available to purchase, from hourly to live-in care for a pre-determined period. Currently, hourly and night-time care is available in London, and live-in care throughout the UK. Once clients input their care needs and what they want (either online or over the phone), Supercarers suggests the kinds of care and carers that might be appropriate.

Many of these start-ups are disrupting the current business model and are yet to prove whether they are viable at scale, but they are a promising sign that new models of providing care and support are being developed.

Not every admission to a care home should be avoided. For some people it provides them with the care and emotional support they need and can be a positive move, particularly for those whose homes are not safe or who have no informal family support. For some the stay is temporary following a health crisis, fall or operation and with the right support and rehabilitation they return home. However, new models of care could help because, simply put, most people don't want to live in a care home. Most of the technology currently being deployed within the care setting is unlikely to be revolutionary and won't replace humans any time soon, but the model of institutional care currently on offer could be significantly disrupted by a growing number of innovative home care models. These offer the hope that it will be possible to provide personalised, family and home-like care to people who need care and support in later life without the negative consequences, either physically or financially, for informal family carers.

The crisis in social care is real, but let's not kid ourselves this is a problem of too many frail older people or people with dementia. Cuts in local authority funding have left many people with no access to services and care providers operating on the edge. In the face of severe cuts and very low fees, local authorities and care providers are doing their best to provide high-quality care. But the situation is critical and unless there is a serious cash injection by the government, as well as a longer-term agreement on how to fund social care, the challenges faced by the care sector will remain. We need to have a serious conversation about what we are willing to pay for a decent social care system. The UK currently spends far too little on social care. We need to fund it properly and do so collectively.

Family carers are already bearing the brunt of these cuts, but they will not be able to fill the gap in care. Unless more is done to value and support carers, fewer people will be willing to provide this vital and yet undervalued personal care and the gap will only get wider. This will require more generous financial support for carers through the benefits system, as well as support for their health and wellbeing, including access to respite care. Otherwise there is a risk that in caring for their loved ones in later life they put their own wellbeing in later life in jeopardy.

It is important we challenge the view that old age is an inevitable time of frailty and decline. Thankfully there are lots of things we know that work to prevent disability and dependency. Key to this is physical activity and in particular activities that increase our muscle strength and improve our balance. It is possible to reverse the loss of function, but this will require a much greater focus on rehabilitation and a change in mindset for us all.

Technology and robots are unlikely to save the day, although they may yet have a role to play. We need to deinstitutionalise care and put in place new models that enable more people with dementia and frailty to live at home or in home-like settings with the care and support they need. If we are to live well at home, with or without the need for care and support, our environment, and in particular the homes we live in, needs to enable us to carry on doing the things we want to do, but as I'll show in the next chapter, housing policy focuses in the wrong place.

8

Home sweet home – or is it?

The current housing crisis is often presented as the fault of the baby boomers, sitting in large properties worth hundreds of thousands of pounds. If only they would downsize, the problem would be solved. Meanwhile younger people, so-called Generation Rent, have no prospect of owning their own home and the lack of social housing means they are at the mercy of rip-off private landlords. Seeing the issue like this has led government to concentrate on first-time buyers, on getting people into the housing market and out of rental, and providing billions in subsidies to house builders, with a focus on quantity not quality.

Planners and developers rarely look at the growing numbers of older households and when they do the typical response is to build specialist housing for those who have care needs or a retirement village that segregates older people from the rest of the community. This failure of imagination and the lack of long-term thinking is creating another less visible housing crisis – one that will condemn people to a lifetime stuck in unsuitable homes that have a negative impact on their health and quality of life. In this chapter I consider how our homes need to change to respond to the age shift.

WHO IS TO BLAME FOR THE HOUSING CRISIS?

The doom-mongers are right to say there is a crisis in our housing market. It is a widely held view. Ipsos Mori found that 79% of adults agree that even if today's young people work hard and get good jobs, they will still have a hard time finding the right housing.[1] The problems appear evident – young people unable to afford to buy a property stuck at home living with their parents, soaring rents consuming a growing proportion of people's income and growing numbers of people homeless, in temporary accommodation, sofa surfing or on the streets – but what is causing these problems?

Let's look first at the evidence on home ownership to understand how this differs by age. Home ownership rates are higher among older age groups. The majority of people 65 years and over are owner-occupiers. In 2017, more than 5.3 million heads of household aged 65 and over owned their own homes (79%). This compares to 57% of those aged 35-44 and 73% of those aged 55-64.[2] To get a fairer comparison we need to look at home ownership rates *at the same age* for different groups born in the same period. According to the Resolution Foundation, in analysis conducted for its Intergenerational Commission, millennials (born between 1981-2000) are half as likely to own a home at age 30 as someone born between 1946 and 1965. However, home ownership rates have been on the decline since those born in the 1940s turned 30. We worry about the millennials, but those born in the 1960s also experienced a decline in home ownership compared to the generation before them. It is possible the situation will change and some of the younger generation will buy a property, albeit at older ages, but the challenge here will be if they then continue to have mortgages to pay later in life.

It does appear that there has been a decline in home ownership. Property has also become concentrated in the hands of fewer people. There has been an increase in both the number of buy-to-let properties and second homes: there were 1.9 million and 1.4 million respectively in Great Britain in 2014-2016, up from 1.2 million buy-to-let properties and 1 million second homes in 2008-2010. Favourable incentives and easy access to buy-to-let mortgages fuelled a huge increase in second properties as investments, particularly among the richer. Analysis from the Resolution Foundation estimates the number of buy-to-let mortgages has risen 15-fold since 2000. In terms of household income distribution, the top fifth of the population owns 67% of the buy-to-let properties and 56% of second homes.[3] Reforms such as removing the tax relief on second property mortgages, reducing (or removing) Council Tax discounts and increasing Stamp Duty on second properties have been introduced to try and solve the problem. While these increase the costs of owning these properties, they don't necessarily make them any more affordable for first-time buyers.

Home ownership is also becoming concentrated in fewer and fewer families, and there is a risk that home ownership becomes the exclusive right of the children or grandchildren of the financially better off and will only increase inequalities among future generations. Indeed, we already see that the children of parents who own property are now three times more likely to become homeowners as the children of those with no property and this gap has widened since the 1990s.[4] The biggest barrier to getting on the housing ladder is a deposit. For many the so-called 'bank of mum and dad' is the only realistic prospect of becoming a homeowner. In 2018, 316,000 people were helped to buy homes by family or friends, supporting the purchase of housing worth £82 billion.[5] In 2016, accounting services company PricewaterhouseCoopers estimated that for a 20- to 39-year-old on an average income looking to buy their first home, it will take nearly two decades (19 years) to save the £115,000 average deposit that will be required to buy a property in 2035, assuming no family help. In 1990, it would have taken the average earner a little over two years.[6] It was my inheritance from my grandfather that enabled me to afford the deposit on my first flat (now nearly 20 years ago), but holding out for the inheritance does not appear to be a good strategy for younger people wanting to secure a deposit on a house. Given life expectancy increases, it is estimated that the most common age at which 20- to 35-year-olds today will inherit will be 61![7]

The two main solutions currently offered to the housing crisis are to get baby boomers to downsize and to subsidise first-time buyers to make buying a property more affordable. Will these strategies work?

WHY DON'T THE BABY BOOMERS DOWNSIZE?

Older homeowners are blamed for 'bedroom blocking' by sitting on assets and not selling up and downsizing. According to the English Housing Survey in 2014-2015, more than half (51%) of older households (classified as occupied by someone over 55) are under-occupied, compared to 23% of younger households.[8] Under-occupancy is defined as having two or more bedrooms that are not required. It is based on assumptions about the number of rooms needed given the age, sex and relationship of the household members; for example, that a couple only uses one bedroom.

However, this measure doesn't take into account how these rooms are actually being used. Sleep problems become more common at older ages and couples may often choose to sleep in separate bedrooms. They might use extra rooms for hobbies or work, or to have friends and family, such as grandchildren, to stay. If the person develops care needs, they may need an extra room in future to provide accommodation for a sleep-in carer. There are a number of reasons why what might be objectively measured as under-occupied is actually fully utilised. While there may be older homeowners with genuinely 'spare' rooms that are surplus to requirements, this is ultimately a decision for the person and not something that can be judged by simply counting the number of rooms in the house. Let's look further into whether people are moving at older ages and, if so, whether they are downsizing?

Overall, people are less likely to move at older ages. Only 3.4% of people aged 50 and over move to a new house every year in the UK. This is half as many moves as the rest of the population. According to research by Manchester School of Architecture, there are currently two main groups of older people who move: 'availability-driven' movers, whose needs are based on aspiration and who want to find suitable housing to meet that aspiration as best they can; and 'accessibility-driven' movers, who move because of problems or lifestyle changes that mean they cannot stay where they were.[9] Those who move by choice generally move at younger ages (50s and 60s) and, while people of all ages move in a crisis or because of a health issue, there is a higher proportion of these types of move at older ages (80s). Those aged 70-74 are least likely to move.

There are many factors that influence an older person's decision about whether to move or not, including emotional attachment to the family home, proximity to family or friends, weighing up the costs and benefits of moving, and the effort or support available to make a move, including decluttering. The favourite policy solution to encourage more older people to move is to abolish Stamp Duty at older ages, but this misses the point, because it assumes older homeowners want to move, but are prevented from doing so simply because of the costs of moving.

Much debate and policy has focused on encouraging older homeowners to downsize, but a 2017 survey by the University of Cambridge showed that, of people over 55 who had recently purchased a home, only 39% had actually downsized; the majority had moved to a house the same size or bigger. One of the key reasons for moving given by people over 55 is the better state of repair and suitability of the new property, by which they mean things like whether or not there are steps.[10] Moving to a smaller property is more common over the age of 80 and is more commonly done by people in social or private rental accommodation. We need to shift the debate from downsizing to 'right-sizing'. 'Right-sizing' is defined as 'an older person's active, positive choice to move home as a means of improving their quality of life'.[11] Jeremy Porteus, a leading housing expert whom I spoke to about these issues, argued that the term needs to be even more aspirational than right-sizing. He proposed the term 'life-seizing' to convey that this is 'about grabbing hold of what our opportunities are, about seeing this as a lifestyle move and much more than the bricks and mortar, but as much about the neighbourhood or community you want to be part of.' I'll come back to looking at the importance of the communities in which we age later in the book.

The lack of movement in the housing market at older ages (other than in a crisis) is not going to be fixed by abolishing Stamp Duty. At least for the next 20 to 30 years there will be demand from older homeowners to right-size to similar size homes. If we are to get people to move before they reach a crisis, these homes will need to offer the possibility of maintaining or improving quality of life rather than being 'the last move'. There is currently a gap in the market across all tenures – i.e. for ownership, private or social rent – of suitable (and affordable) options. Homes are not available in the right place, of the right size, nor are they accessible or adaptable to enable people to have a better quality of life into old age. As we will see later in the chapter, we must not only build more homes, we must also build the right homes.

HELPING FIRST-TIME BUYERS

The second focus of current policy is to make new homes more affordable to first-time buyers. National planning rules now require a proportion of new builds to be 'affordable'. The government also provides subsidies to first-time buyers through the Help to Buy scheme, which provides a five-year, interest-free loan of up to 20% of the cost of a newly built home (40% in London), effectively enabling those without access to family wealth to pay a deposit and get on the housing ladder. Shared ownership is the other government-backed scheme which means the new property is jointly owned with a housing association. The individual purchases between 25% and 75% of the property and pays rent on the rest (except those over the age of 55 who, if they own 75%, don't pay rent). The Help to Buy scheme has so far given out 211,000 loans at a cost of £11.7 billion to the taxpayer since it was introduced in 2013.[12] While 37% of buyers said they could not have bought a house without the loan, one-fifth of the loans were to people who already owned property.

While these schemes may have helped some people to buy a home who could otherwise not have afforded to do so, in those parts of the country with very high house prices, they do not make a home truly affordable if measured against earnings (rather than against relative house prices). The cost of buying a home has risen at twice the rate of general inflation, so that on average a home in England costs eight times average earnings.[13]

These schemes also don't touch the buying and selling of existing homes. Even if the baby boomers were to move and sell up, these homes are unlikely to be affordable to first-time buyers, particularly without the subsidies available when they purchase a new build. There has also been growth in the build-to-rent market, but these schemes don't address the affordability of rents either (an issue I will come back to later in the chapter).

If we want housing to be available and more affordable for people of all ages, we need to stop blaming the baby boomers and focus on the real problem: lack of supply.

WHY WE NEED TO BUILD MORE HOMES

Supply of housing has not kept pace with demand. Between 1996 and 2014, the number of households in the UK grew from 23.7 million to 26.7 million.[14] While in theory we have built enough homes to accommodate this growth (3.3 million homes over the same period[15]), we have not recognised the changing composition of households. Many more people are living in one- or two-person households. After the 2008 recession, the overall number of houses built dropped below 200,000 a year, which some believe is the minimum needed to keep up with population growth.[16] Since the 1950s Germany has built twice as many homes as the UK and even this is perceived to fall short of what is needed. While Germany builds at a rate of more than 3 homes for every 1000 people each year, the UK builds less than 2.7 homes per 1000.[17] However, privately financed house building has continued (2.7 million homes since 1996[18]) and the significant gap is due to the lack of local authority investment in new homes in recent years (see graph on page 207).

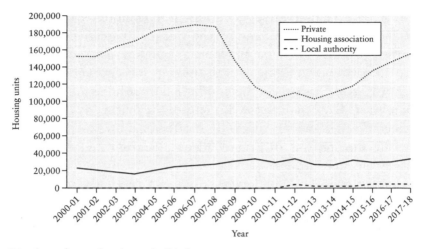

Number of completed new builds by tenure.

Source: Ministry of Housing, Communities and Local Government, Live tables on house building: new build dwellings (2019).

In 2012, local authorities were subjected to a limit on the amount of money they could borrow to fund social housing and this stymied any investment in building new council homes. This cap was lifted in October 2018 and according to the OBR it is expected that this will increase house building by about 4,000 new homes a year, resulting in 20,000 more council housing by 2023-2024.[19] However, while Right to Buy (introduced in the 1980s, giving council tenants the right to purchase the property they rent at a substantially discounted rate) remains in place, this growth in new building is unlikely to result in a huge increase in the total number of homes actually available for social rent, as they will simply replace the units sold. In contrast, social housing providers have been able to borrow capital, but have faced other constraints, including the availability of financial subsidies to build affordable homes for shared ownership schemes. Some developments have included homes for sale privately in order to subsidise the social and affordable housing schemes, but demand for these private properties collapsed following the financial crisis in 2008, resulting in a reduction in the number of homes being built by both social and private developers in 2010-2011.

The last Conservative government committed to building 300,000 new homes a year by the mid-2020s with the aim of boosting home ownership. House builders and developers are focused on building starter homes for first-time buyers, because, as we have seen, this is where the subsidies are targeted. Developers like building for this end of the market as these sales can go through quickly as they are often chain free – people are usually moving out of rented accommodation and provide a steady pipeline of sales.

But the big house builders are missing a trick. Already almost one third of all English households are occupied *exclusively* by people age 55 and over – over 7 million households – and most of these are owner-occupiers.[20] The number of older households is set to increase rapidly in the next 25 years. Households headed by someone aged 65 years and over are expected to increase by 3.5 million from 28% of all households in England in 2016 to 37% in 2041. The proportion of households over 85 years old is projected to double over the same time period.[21] We must build homes for people of all ages.

As the UK embarks on a major house-building programme, as it must, how can we ensure that these homes are fit for an ageing population?

WHAT SORT OF HOUSING DO WE NEED TO BUILD?

We have an opportunity with the prospect of a major building boom to get these homes right for generations to come and to build homes that will enable the 1960s baby boomers to live in homes that will allow them to remain active and independent for longer.

Currently, if planners and developers think about housing for an ageing population, they immediately think of *specialist* housing, that is, homes that are designed and marketed for older people. Such developments often come with some sort of care available if needed or are part of a retirement community with other facilities on site. Needless to say, given the age shift, there probably needs to be more of this, too, but this will more likely appeal to people in that phase of dependency towards the end of life or those forced to make a 'crisis' move. There are often service charges (sometimes very high ones) that people are reluctant to pay, particularly if they don't actually need the extra care on offer. Even among those 70 years old and older who move to a new house, only one in four moves into specialist housing.[22] And around 90% of people aged 50 and over live in mixed communities and general needs housing. So, if this is not just about building specialist homes for old people, how can we ensure homes are built in mixed-age developments that will last a lifetime? The solution must be to require all new homes to be built to higher accessibility standards.

The Joseph Rowntree Foundation, an independent charity that is focused on poverty but has historically worked to improve the quality of housing for older people, introduced the idea of the lifetime home in the early 1990s (see box on page 210). Since then the concept has developed into a standard based on 16 design features that make a dwelling adaptable as the circumstances and mobility of the occupant changes.

These standards are compulsory in a few places, but a lack of data means we don't know how many homes are built to the standards and if you're looking to buy a property it's also hard to find out which standards they meet. This suggests the need for a rating similar to the energy ratings listed when a property is for sale. Current national government guidelines require that all new homes must meet Category M I standards for accessibility. These require homes to have four basic features so that people with different needs can visit them: level access at the front door, flush thresholds, wide doorframes and a toilet at entrance level. This simply means that an elderly relative with mobility issues could come and visit, but not stay overnight. Standards should be set higher (Category M II), so that all new houses are also built to be flexible and adaptable to enable someone with a mobility issue to live there, for example, by providing a larger space on the entrance level that could accommodate a bathroom as well as a toilet. This would mean that people would be able to put in aids and adaptations like grab rails or wet rooms when they need them without huge cost or difficulty.

THE 16 DESIGN FEATURES OF A LIFETIME HOME

Lifetime homes have to be built to very specific technical standards developed by a group of housing experts, which I won't go in to here. I will, however, list the factors that have to be considered when building to that standard.

1 Car parking width
2 Access from car parking
3 Approach gradients to entrances
4 Entrance space and design
5 Communal stairs and lifts
6 Doorways and hallways
7 Wheelchair accessibility
8 Entrance-level living room
9 Entrance-level bedspace
10 Entrance-level WC and shower drainage
11 Bathroom and WC walls
12 Stair lift/through-floor lift
13 Tracking hoist route
14 Bathroom layout
15 Window specification
16 Location of service controls

Source: Lifetime Homes Foundation, *Lifetime Homes Standard*, revised (2010).

Local authorities are responsible for developing local plans that influence what sorts of houses are built and where. Some forward-thinking authorities like the Greater London Authority (GLA) are thinking differently about the housing needs of the future and have introduced local requirements that all new homes have to meet higher accessibility standards than the minimum required. Other councils that have tried to require all new homes to be built to higher accessibility standards have met with objections from the house builders, primarily on cost grounds, even though the additional cost at the building stage is modest. It is estimated to cost just £521 in building costs to meet Category M II standards for a three-bedroom property and a further £1,000 for the additional space requirements compared to Category M I. This is very similar to estimates of the additional costs of building to lifetime standards (which are slightly different) at the design stage, which were estimated at £1,500.[23]

Building accessible homes at the beginning is much cheaper than adapting them later. The average amount for a Disabled Facilities Grant, which local authorities give to people on low incomes to help with the cost of adapting their home for things such as adding grab rails or widening doorways, is £9,000, but the cost of major adaptations can reach £30,000.[24] We should really be thinking about the costs over the lifetime of the home.

Developers also argue that there is a lack of demand for accessible housing and that adding further cost to homebuilding will prevent young families getting on to the housing ladder, though it's hard to see that £1,500 is really going to make a difference to affordability. However, an accessible home with wider doorways and entrance-level facilities is not just useful for older or disabled occupants, but also parents with prams, anyone carrying luggage or with temporarily restricted mobility, for example, due to a sports injury. Given the lack of mobility in the housing market, people are less likely to move as often and so the homes people are buying in early stages of their lives will ideally need to meet their changing needs throughout their lives.

Inclusively designed and accessible homes could transform the lives of millions of older people today and in future generations. The government could very easily require all new developments to meet higher accessibility standards. Without this, local authorities, particularly those in areas where there is low demand, will continue to face opposition from developers and only the most forward-thinking developers (both in the social and private sector) will voluntarily build to the higher standards. Without a level playing field they are unlikely to see this as making business sense, particularly where the standards increase the space requirements, thereby reducing the number of units they can fit on the same plot of land.

My own parents are in their late 70s and thankfully remain fit and active. They live in a tall Victorian terrace, so get plenty of exercise going up and down stairs. While they manage these now, I worry what will happen if a sudden deterioration in their health leaves them less mobile. A fall down the stone steps to the cellar, which in winter they use daily to fetch coal and logs for the open fire, would be catastrophic. I see the risks, but for them it's their home. They fitted a handrail beside the cellar steps some years ago and this has helped when carrying heavy loads up the steps and helping balance on the way down.

They plan to move sometime, but I sense that my mother is reluctant due to her emotional ties to her childhood home. She lived there as a child and they have enjoyed living there for nearly 50 years! They have been amazing at decluttering – often a major impediment to people moving in later life. While the town does have a high-end retirement village with social facilities on site and the option of care if needed, this isn't centrally located and is not attractive to my parents, who have friends of all ages and are very involved in the life of the town.

Generally, there are options for those at the extreme ends of the socio-economic gradient. The very wealthy can afford to seek out 'premium' retirement developments (built to accessible standards, but don't necessarily go beyond the minimum requirements). Those without assets will theoretically be supported by the state to move into accessible or sheltered housing. The challenge is that the average social housing tenant is already quite old – nearly a third of social renters are over 65[25] – and not all social housing is suitable for older people to live in, suggesting there needs to be investment in new social housing that meets the needs of existing and future older tenants.

Jeremy Porteus, a leading expert on housing for older people, believes the real challenges lie with those on low to middle incomes, particularly for low-income homeowners. He observed that some of these people exercised their right to buy, under Thatcher's government 30 or 40 years ago and now find it difficult to maintain their properties. They don't have the equity either to afford a more accessible property in the same area. Those who only part-own their property or have short leaseholds may find it difficult to sell or have insufficient equity to buy. He argues that there is a real gap in the market for major financial institutions to come up with more consumer-savvy products for homeowners – on trusted terms rather than the current equity release and lifetime mortgages – to benefit this group of people. While much of the emphasis has been on the first-time buyer with 'help to buy' products, he suggests new 'help to retire' products are needed which could safeguard the quality of accommodation as we age, for example, having a maintenance contract or insurance as part of the loan to ensure the property is maintained while the person is living in it.

It will be critical for both private housing developers, as well as local authorities and social housing providers, to recognise the importance of all homes being built to these accessibility standards. Given the shortages of land for building in many towns and cities, and the protection of green belt in rural areas, this is unlikely to mean everyone living in bungalows. We need architects and designers to think more innovatively about how to make accessible homes attractive for people of all ages and how to reduce the costs of building these homes further. I'll look at some current innovations in the final section of this chapter.

However, even if all new homes are built to be accessible, the fact is that most of the homes we will live in over the next 50 years are already built. So what needs to be done to make sure these homes are safe and accessible for the growing number of older households?

UPGRADING EXISTING HOUSING

Over 80% of older people say they want to stay in their own home as they age[26] and our homes are where we spend a lot of time, particularly as we get older. The condition and design of the house can therefore make a big difference to our health and quality of life, and yet the UK has the oldest housing stock in the European Union, with more than a third (36%) of the existing housing stock having been built before 1946.[27]

The focus of health and care policy has tended to be on keeping people in their homes for longer and 'maintaining independence'. This reflects the concerns of service providers and funders about the high costs of residential and nursing care if people have to be admitted to an institutional setting. But we must challenge the idea of 'ageing in place' if this means remaining in the same home even if it's to the detriment of health or quality of life. The focus needs to be on the person and whether the home environment enables people to live the life they want to lead day to day. While, for some, their home can be adapted or they can use aids and assistive technologies, for others, it would be better to move home (despite the upheaval) to somewhere that is safe and free from hazards, warm, dry and well insulated, that is designed to be accessible or easily adapted. So what is the state of existing housing and what needs to be done to make it fit for the future?

GETTING THE BASICS RIGHT: MAKING HOMES WARM AND SAFE

Poor housing conditions can have a direct negative impact on our health. Our homes can also be hazardous, resulting in dangerous trips, slips and falls. Home hazards such as excess cold, excess heat, damp, asbestos, fire hazards, overcrowding and disrepair all contribute directly to a lack of health, safety and wellbeing.[28] The most recent comprehensive survey of older people's housing conditions in 2014[29] found that as many as one in five homes

(20%) occupied by people over 55 in England (that's equivalent to 2 million households) failed the Decent Homes Standard. These standards require homes to be free of hazards (such as a leaking roof or a broken boiler that could cause damage to health or injury) and in a reasonable state of repair, and for the facilities to be reasonably modern (for example, a kitchen that has been modernised in the last 20 years and a bathroom that's less than 30 years old), and for the home to provide a reasonable level of warmth. Those aged 85 years or over were more likely to live in non-decent housing (29%) compared with all other age groups. Across all age groups, almost 3 million homes in England had at least one so-called category 1 hazard (a hazard that poses a serious and immediate risk to a person's health and safety), and around 1.3 million of these were in homes occupied by households aged 55 years and over.[30] This is shocking and needs to be addressed, not only for the sake of the people who live in these places, but also to reduce the huge costs to society.

The state of our housing adds to the pressures on the NHS. Economic analysis by the Building Research Establishment, an independent building science centre, has estimated the cost of poor housing to the NHS alone to be £1.4 billion per annum, equivalent to that of alcohol or smoking. In this analysis, cold homes and fall hazards contributed by far the largest proportion of those costs, with the risk of fires and hazards caused by damp the next most significant causes of health costs. If all fall hazards were fixed, this could save the NHS £435 million per year.[31]

Poor quality housing is not distributed evenly across the country or by tenure. Non-decent homes are more likely to be concentrated in industrial cities in the North. A recent report by a consortium of housing providers in the north of England found that a third of England's non-decent homes are concentrated in the North, many in the North West. More than a quarter (26%) of non-decent homes in the North West are owner-occupied. Official estimates suggest that the cost of repairing the one million non-decent owner-occupied homes in the North would be nearly £8 billion, far exceeding costs in the rest of the country.[32]

A major investment programme in social housing means that the majority of these properties are 'decent', although social housing providers should not be complacent about the ongoing need for investment in upgrading older properties. Older low-income homeowners and private renters are more likely to be living in poor quality housing. A major issue is that homeowners who were once able to maintain their homes themselves, doing DIY and repairs when they were working and fitter, are now unable to do them and can no longer afford to pay tradespeople for one-off repairs and maintenance costs, because they rely on a state pension or a small private pension. Local authority grants do exist for improving the condition of homes, but due to local authority funding these have reduced drastically and only those in receipt of benefits or Pension Credit are likely to receive them.[33]

Some homeowners take a loan out against the equity in their property in order to fund home renovations. However, some vulnerable owner-occupiers may need additional support to manage the building works. Legal and General, a leading financial services company, which offers an equity release product, teamed up with the London Rebuilding Society, a social enterprise organisation working to improve housing conditions for homeowners over 55, to provide an end-to-end home improvement scheme – decluttering properties, rehousing people while work is done, specifying and managing the works, identifying and overseeing contractors, and supporting the person to move back in at the end. Such a bespoke service is neither needed nor affordable for everyone. However, there are likely to be many people who, if they could access some support as well as the finances, would be able to make changes to their home more easily.

Older and poorer households are much more likely to be living in unsafe conditions. Shelter and security are basic needs. It is shocking that in 21st-century Britain we still tolerate older people living in such poor housing conditions. While there are several discretionary funds available, because of cuts in the direct grant from national government to local councils these have been routinely diverted for other purposes. Providing adequate funding to local government or creating new ring-fenced capital grants for low-income homeowners to make repairs to their home may be part of the answer, together with tighter regulation of private landlords who fail to meet standards and tougher enforcement. However, nothing short of a major upgrade in the existing housing stock is needed if we want to ensure that everyone can live in a home that is warm and safe into old age.

FUTURE-PROOFING: MAKING HOMES ACCESSIBLE AND ADAPTABLE

Not only are some homes in a shocking state of repair, they are also poorly designed. The best source of data is the English Housing Survey and it found that 93% of homes lack the four basic features that deem them 'visitable' by disabled people[34], including step free access at the front of the house, a level access at the front door, wide doors and a downstairs toilet. Some homes can easily be adapted, but the age and condition of the housing in the UK – think of the rows of Victorian terraces with steps up to the front door and steep stairs inside – means the vast majority of our existing housing stock is unfit for us as we age. According to Jeremy Porteus, the housing expert, 'The biggest challenge we face is the lack of adaptable housing,' especially as most of the housing older people and those approaching later life live in was built in the last 150 years and is 'past their sell-by date'.

For some older people with disabilities, houses are so poorly designed that they find themselves prisoners in their own homes. And yet this could be so different. Even very simple changes to our homes can make a big difference to our ability to manage daily activities, such as washing and bathing, but getting access to adaptations is difficult. There are often long waits to be assessed, funding is means tested, and aids and adaptations that are available to buy direct are often unattractive and only available in specialist shops.

Obtaining an estimate of the number of people needing adaptations is difficult. The English Housing Survey shows that around 18% of households headed by an adult aged 65 or over lack one or more of the adaptations they require, such as a grab rail or adapted shower room. This is highly likely to be an underestimate as it relies on self-reporting and evidence is clear that people tend to under-report their support needs. We know that if adaptations are completed in good time, alongside any necessary repairs and with the individual's personal goals in mind, they can improve a range of health and wellbeing outcomes for people in later life.[35]

When people's abilities change, if their environment is not adapted it can result in a severe reduction in quality of life. One woman interviewed as part of a study of home adaptations had lost mobility, couldn't use the stairs and didn't have a loo downstairs, so began restricting her intake of liquids so she didn't need to go to the toilet. She ended up crawling upstairs on her hands and knees.[36] Such situations should not be acceptable in a civilised society. Lack of a well-designed environment can be disabling. Take someone with limited mobility and reduced control over their urinary function as an example. In a home where the toilet is up a flight of stairs, they are effectively incontinent, having to use pads as they are unable to get to the toilet in time. The same person living in a home with a ground floor toilet easily and quickly accessible from the kitchen or living room might well find they can successfully get to the toilet.

The design of our homes, and the extent to which they are accessible and adaptable, is also vitally important to keep us socially connected. If our home is badly designed, for example, with lots of steps to the front door, and we have health conditions that limit our ability to move around, such as breathing difficulties or arthritis, we are likely to find it difficult to get out and may become socially isolated.

People with high levels of health needs are entitled to receive a home assessment from an occupational therapist. A good home assessment should look at all aspects of the home – the condition and state of repair, lighting and trip hazards, as well as adaptations – focusing on what the individual, and family carer if relevant, wants to do in their home – what's important to them. Unfortunately, there are long waiting times to be assessed and the quality of assessment varies. Some areas are changing how they do assessments as there simply aren't enough occupational therapists (OTs) to carry them out. Jeremy Porteus suggested OTs could play a role in training and supporting others to make those decisions. He also says it is important that consumers are part of the assessment or could be supported by 'consumers by experience' who themselves have benefited from adaptations. Research by the Centre for Ageing Better has suggested that the best outcomes are achieved when individuals, families and carers are closely involved in the decision-making process, focusing on individual goals and what a person wants to achieve in the home.[37]

Some local areas are trying out new approaches to improve the timeliness and quality of both assessment, and delivery of improvement and adaptation works. For example, in Brent and Brighton, they are training other professionals such as handyperson agencies to carry out minor repairs and adaptations, as well as give advice on fall prevention. In Wigan, the fire service has integrated assessments into its 'safe and well' checks. Targeted at over 65s, these provide advice on slips, trips and falls, as well as signposting people to heart checks and bowel cancer screening. They also offer advice and support on smoking and alcohol consumption. In Sunderland, they have set up a pool of approved contractors to avoid the need to tender for each major job and to co-ordinate the visits of different professionals in order to avoid unnecessary delays. These innovations are fragile, however. They are typically based on small-scale pilots, short-term contracts and stop-start funding, with constant uncertainty for providers and practitioners. These approaches need to be brought together into a much more consistent approach across the country, with much greater integration between housing, the NHS and social care.

There is state funding, called the Disabled Facilities Grant (DFG), to help people on low incomes afford refurbishments and adaptations, but ironically, despite a recent increase in the DFG funding available (£473 million in 2017-2018), this money is not translating into action everywhere, with some councils reporting underspends. There is a backlog of assessments in the system and so local authorities can't get rid of the money fast enough. Means testing also slows things down. Local authorities are now being encouraged to eliminate means testing for some of the cheaper minor adaptations, so that more people benefit. This approach would be of benefit to cash-poor owner-occupiers, who are generally ineligible for grants because of their home ownership, but who do not have the immediate means to pay for improvements themselves.

In comparison to the private sector many social housing providers have schemes to provide modifications and adaptations in a timely way. Durham Housing Group directly funds aids and adaptations for its tenants and employs occupational therapists who assess need, liaise with health and care professionals, and may advise on a move or minor or major adaptations. But where housing associations do make modifications and adaptations, these are frequently removed again when a new tenant moves in. More sophisticated and planned matching of tenants to properties would avoid this unnecessary waste.

There was a recent case I heard about of a couple who had a time-limited leasehold on their property. When their circumstances changed, the freeholder did not allow them to install the necessary adaptations. They took the case to court and the court ruled in the disabled woman's favour, arguing that allowing adaptations was a reasonable adjustment for her disability.

It seems crazy, doesn't it, that there is government funding for adaptations, but not to deal with the basic condition and hazards in the home; that the funding is there for the adaptation, but not to employ people to do the assessment and process the claims; that lots of people could benefit from adaptations who are otherwise stuck in hospital, but there are long waiting times to see OTs to do the assessments. The system is broken and needs a radical overhaul, so that more people get what they need in a timely way.

INCLUSIVE DESIGN FOR THE HOME

Even if this system were fixed, as Jeremy Porteus reminded me, 'The majority of people who make changes to existing homes don't do it through DFG, they just go to the nearest DIY superstore. While it is encouraging to see IKEA is now developing accessible living spaces, we need an urgent rethink on how the retail sector is responding to our ageing population. Twenty years ago when I visited Japan I saw how inclusively designed products were being retailed on the high street. What's the mainstream equivalent here if you want to future-proof your home?'

You'd find that most of the products are ugly and expensive. They are more likely to be sold from an out-of-town industrial unit than on the high street or they can be found on obscure websites for clinical and medical supplies, not on the shelves of IKEA or B&Q. It is little wonder, then, that people are put off installing adaptations in their home for fear of how 'medical' or unattractive they will look. As yet, designers and retailers are not creating or marketing affordable, attractive products to support independent living. Can't we still have taste and style as we grow older?

There is also insufficient awareness among consumers doing up their homes of the potential benefits of adaptations, so they don't demand them. People just aren't aware of some of the changes they could make. For example, putting in a walk-in level-access shower or wetroom, fitting lever door handles rather than knobs and easy-to-use lever taps on sinks, or positioning electric sockets at knee height rather than ankle level. The list goes on.

Products such as grip rails for baths and showers should be designed and supplied as standard along with other bathroom accessories. There are lots of other products or modifications that can be made to homes that would enable people to live independently into old age – features that don't necessarily need special products. Wouldn't it be better if when we were investing

221

in a new kitchen or bathroom – long before we needed it – we were advised to fit an eye-level oven or to create a walk-in shower with attractive fittings that are weight-bearing? This requires a massive shift in the market – in those designing products for the home so they are inclusive, attractive and affordable, in those who are retailing these products to market them to consumers of all ages and abilities, and in the intermediaries such as builders and tradespeople who install and fit them. It will also require us to change. We need to demand these products and think ahead to future-proof our homes.

IS IT THE END OF HOME OWNERSHIP?

We imagine Generation Rent to be those young millennials unable to get on the housing ladder. But the number of older renters is set to increase rapidly, so what does it mean to be part of Generation Rent when you reach your 60s and 70s?

The number of older private renters is small but growing, while the number renting socially has fallen. In 2017, there were 1.1 million (16%) older households renting from a local authority or housing association where the head of household was over 65 years old, a reduction from 1.24 million (25%) in 2003. Just 380,000 (6%) over 65s privately rented in 2017, an increase from 220,000 (4%) in 2003. This is likely to increase in the future: there was a 24% rise in the number of private renters aged 55-64 between 2010 and 2017, and a decline in the proportion who own their own home from 82% in 2003-2004 to 73% in 2017-2018.[38] The proportion of older private renters is growing and one estimate suggests the proportion of households over the age of 64 who are privately renting will increase from 5% now to 12% in 2046, more than doubling.[39] The trends point to a dramatic increase in the number of older private renters in future – people like James, one of the worried and disconnected group from the Later Life Study, who rents his home from the son of his former partner. He is keen to stay in this home for the rest of his life, since it is a bungalow and meets his needs. His friends also live locally, and he is able to drive around and has access to everything he needs. Although he gets on well with his landlord, James' tenancy is still relatively insecure as the rent could increase or his ex-step son could decide to sell up.

So what issues will the increase in older renters raise? First, there is the issue of affordability. Older private renters may struggle financially, particularly if they are on a fixed pension income and rents are increased. As we saw in the chapter on money, most calculations for the amount of savings people need in retirement are calculated after housing costs, so those with only modest pensions could struggle to pay their rent. Those without savings who rely solely on the state pension and are in receipt of Pension Credit are able to claim Housing Benefit, a personal subsidy which enables non-working households and those on a low income to pay for rented accommodation. Currently 1.25 million of the 4.2 million Housing Benefit claimants are over 65, costing the state approximately £6 billion per year.[40] Estimates by the Resolution Foundation suggest that in the most pessimistic scenario it modelled, where only 66% of millennials own their own home in retirement, the bill could reach as much as £16 billion in 2060.[41] While it is paid to both social and private landlords, social rents are usually set at 50% of market rents. Since 2011 social housing providers have also offered 'affordable' rents at 80% of market value.

Second, private renters move more frequently than people in other tenures. Private renters in the 50-69 age group are over three times more likely to move than those who own or socially rent their homes, with 14% moving every year.[42] These frequent moves are also likely to be disruptive, potentially affecting someone's ability to work, to access local services and informal support in their local community, and disrupting the social networks that are so important to the wellbeing of older people. Some of these moves may be 'forced' due to the lack of security of tenure, particularly under the assured shorthold tenancy agreements that mean landlords can give notice and require people to move out.

This is also a factor in the growth in homelessness. In 2015-2016, a third of all households that were made homeless were put in this situation due to the ending of an assured shorthold tenancy. Some of the other reasons for people becoming homeless at older ages include family breakdown and redundancy. It is also possible that other sudden changes in circumstances, such as bereavement or inability to work due to poor health or disability, could result in a change in finances and an inability to keep up with rent. There has been a huge increase in the numbers of homeless people over the age of 60. According to Shelter, the homelessness charity, 2,520 people aged 60 and over were accepted as homeless in 2017-2018 – a staggering rise of 40% in the last five years and the highest number for over a decade.[43] This rise in homelessness at older ages is a worrying trend.

Third, private renters may find it more difficult to adapt their homes to meet their needs. There is no requirement for landlords to agree to adaptations or changes in the building, although they cannot unreasonably withhold consent. Also, in order to receive the funding available for those on low incomes to adapt their home (via the DFG), applicants must intend to be in the property for at least five years to be eligible. As a result, those in private rental are much less likely to be recipients of DFG funding and only around 7% of all grants go to private renters[44] although they account for 19% of the market.[45]

Finally, private rented accommodation is more likely to be cold and damp, and therefore hazardous to health, because as we've seen, private rented accommodation has the highest proportion of 'non-decent' homes compared to owner-occupied homes and social rented homes.

A number of changes are needed in order to ensure those who enter later life who don't own their own home are able to live safely and independently. There needs to be stronger landlord regulation and better use made of local authority enforcement powers. Increasing numbers of local authorities have introduced standards and require landlords with certain types of housing to apply for a license. However, they have limited capacity to enforce those standards and there is very little evaluation of the difference these powers are making. Liverpool is the only city to have implemented the scheme city-wide (since 2015) and this has been subject to legal challenges by landlords. Better regulation of landlords and protections for tenants would not only tackle the problems faced by older private renters but would help Generation Rent to access high-quality rented accommodation and enjoy greater security of tenure.

As well, central government needs to increase the public funding available to local authorities to invest in the renewal of properties, including re-instating funding for private sector renewal. Investing in upgrading the condition of properties would mean they were cheaper to heat and maintain and could reduce costs to the NHS in the long term. This would have a wider public benefit. Alternatively, we need new social financing methods to create the upfront investment in housing renewal to generate these longer-term returns. In Hull, a charity called Giroscope has secured investment to renovate properties in the city, which is generating both a financial and a social return (see box below).

GIROSCOPE – RENOVATING HOMES IN HULL

Giroscope is a community charity based in Hull. It was set up in the mid-1980s with the aim of tackling the city's poor supply of privately rented housing. As well as low standards in the rented sector, industrial decline had also led to low levels of owner-occupation and a significant number of vacant properties.

Giroscope buys and renovates empty properties to provide housing for those in need, utilising a large volunteer force, many of whom are at risk of social exclusion, including young people, those who are unemployed and homeless people. Prospective tenants are also able to help with renovation projects.

By 2017, Giroscope owned nearly a hundred properties, housing more than 250 people, mostly in west Hull. This number has grown recently, with the support of two investments, in 2015 and 2017, from Social and Sustainable Capital, a social investor that invests in charities and social enterprises.

We also need to reform tenancies to address the limited means of complaint and redress available to tenants and reduce the prevalence of short-term tenancies. The landlord-tenant relationship in the UK is archaic and the rights of tenants need to be strengthened, with longer and more secure tenancies made available. We would do well to learn from countries like Germany where long-term lease arrangements are much more common, where the tenant has more of stake in the property and there is a strong social contract. The government consulted on introducing three-year tenancies in 2018, but dropped these proposals after opposition. The Tenant Fees Act, which came into force in mid-2019, made limited reforms to introduce lower maximum deposits and curtail letting agent fees, but it fell far short of what is needed to protect private renters, young and old.

Finally, we need to expand social housing and make it easier for older private renters to transfer tenures. Social landlords can provide more affordable options and more secure tenancies. Indeed, lifetime tenancies are still the norm, although the government has allowed social housing providers to offer fixed-term tenancies since 2012, usually of five years. However, many older people do not know they might be eligible for social housing, depending on their level of need. While not being able to access your home due to a disability is likely to make someone a high priority for council housing, if they have made themselves 'intentionally homeless', for example, by leaving a property because they are in either rent or mortgage arrears but before they were evicted, they could be considered to have left voluntarily. There is also a stigma associated with social housing that needs addressing if older people who have lived in private rented accommodation, or homeowners who cannot afford to maintain their property, are to be encouraged to move. However, this will require a major expansion in new homes being built for social rent. There are 2 million fewer homes owned by housing associations and local authorities than there were in 1980. The number of new units built for social rent also declined from 39,560 in 2010-2011 to just 6,463 in 2017-2018. After the introduction of 'affordable' rents, the number built for social rent rapidly grew to 40,830 new units in 2014-2015,[46] but there is still a significant shortfall and long waiting lists indicate that demand far exceeds availability.

So, while home ownership at older ages is high, we can expect the rates to fall year on year and to see an increase in the number of older renters. The decline in the availability of social housing means that the proportion of those in the private rented sector will increase. Many of the policies which would benefit Generation Rent – such as landlord licensing to improve the condition of private rented accommodation, secure and longer-term tenancies, and affordable rents – would obviously also make a huge difference to the outcomes for renters at older ages. And social housing needs to invest in remodelling existing stock and building new stock to meet the needs not only of their existing tenants, but also to extend social rent to pensioners switching from other tenures. This would benefit both the individual, who would benefit from security of tenure and more affordable rents, and the state, which would save on Housing Benefit. Responding to this will require investment in new accessible and affordable homes across all tenures, but rather than just build more of the same we need to be more imaginative in thinking about the homes of the future.

NEW MODELS FOR LIVING – HOMES OF THE FUTURE

There is huge interest in how technology will transform the way we live. Can smart homes not only be energy-efficient, but also enable us to continue to live independently at older ages? There is already a lot of everyday technology that can be used to assist with daily living and new advances in robotics are set to change this further. When I visited the New Old exhibition at the Design

Museum in London I saw a serviced apartment with hidden service corridors where people (or robots) could replenish your fridge or return your fresh laundry without ever having contact with you. A world in which you would never need to leave your flat but would also not see the people who came to help you felt dystopian, although it may not be far from reality if we do nothing, as we'll see in the final chapter.

As we saw in the previous chapter on care, telehealth and telecare products are already widely used to support people to manage their long-term conditions and to monitor people in their homes. They often use a combination of personal and environmental sensors to monitor the safety and wellbeing of older people in their own homes. They are connected to remote monitoring, in the case of telehealth to a clinical care team who will be alerted if there are any worrying changes in the person's vital signs, and in the case of telecare it might be to a family member or carer who will be alerted if there have been any changes, for example, someone going to the toilet in the night but not returning to bed, indicating they might have fallen.

Smart homes – the idea that the Internet of Things together with sensors and other connectivity can allow you to autonomously control, for example, the temperature or lighting – is also becoming a reality and could be used to ensure that those with cognitive decline, mobility or health conditions are able to live safely by, say, adjusting the temperature or turning off cookers when the meal is ready.

New construction techniques also open up opportunities for alternative approaches to accessible homes. The return of modular homes, such as those being manufactured by Legal and General (see box opposite) creates new opportunities to build in inclusive and accessible design features, and to produce homes more efficiently, thereby making them more affordable. It may also be easier to build in modular features, such as movable walls that can create bigger rooms if someone needs additional equipment, from the start.

NEW CONSTRUCTION TECHNIQUES

Large-scale investment in modular housing, much of the construction of which can be done in a factory at a much quicker speed than traditional housebuilding, has been billed as a possible solution to the UK's housebuilding shortfall.

In 2017, insurance company Legal and General released its first prototype modular home, which is mostly constructed off-site. The company hopes that within four years it will be able to produce more than 3,000 of these homes at its factory in Yorkshire and build and install them at sites around the UK. In the factory, all homes are fitted with kitchens, bathrooms, electrics, plumbing and internal decoration, meaning that only cladding, roofing and some internal works need to be done on site.

Modular homes are much cheaper to make and to maintain. The aim is that they will also be cheaper to buy and rent and be a more affordable option for those who cannot buy traditionally built homes. In December 2018, Legal and General delivered its first modular homes to a site near Bracknell in Berkshire.

Self-build is also increasingly popular and together with new construction methods could make it more economical to design customised homes, thus enabling smaller plots of land to be utilised to provide accessible homes close to where people live, for example, in-fill sites. Design prizes could stimulate new homes that are cheap and efficient to build, that meet high environmental standards and are accessible – the green lifetime home.

It is also likely that there will be new ownership models for later life living. There has been major investment in many city centres in large modern blocks for rent. Originally designed as student accommodation, developers quickly recognised there was demand for flats for young professionals just starting out.

These rental properties are managed by large management companies and tend to have better standards of maintenance and safety (partly because they are new, and partly because of the business model and level of rent). Jeremy Porteus is interested in this model for older renters. He believes there is growing interest from developers in something that is closer to a model of licensed residential care, where you separate out the lodgings and care and, in some cases, there may not really be care at all. Developers are offering longer tenancies, such as a seven-year fixed tenancy, and different models of tenure, which are better than six-month or one-year tenancies. Given the predicted rise in private renting, a greater diversity of options is needed to provide security of tenure, as well as homes that are safe, well maintained and affordable. Shared ownership is also becoming more common and could open up opportunities for low income homeowners without the equity to afford to buy outright to move to a more suitable home in later life, which they would part-own, particularly given that, under the current government's Older People's Shared Ownership (OPSO) scheme, over 55s who own up to 75% of the property don't pay rent on the rest.

The final area of innovation is models of shared or communal forms of living. I asked Jeremy Porteus what he thought we should be building in terms of housing for the future. He said there was a need to think about different types of collaborative housing to achieve greater community and personal resilience, such as co-housing and co-living. He explained that this could be age-designated or intergenerational. Co-living includes shared communal facilities, like kitchens and lounges, with each person having their own living unit. Co-housing is usually more stable communities where the residents have their own private homes in addition to shared facilities, for example, a guest room. As well as relying on each other for help and support, some of the co-housing residents can then share additional services like a gardener, handyman or carer if they develop care and support needs.

Could these new models of shared living provide a better solution to underfunded care homes? I, for one, would rather live with my friends in a co-housing development and club together to pay for care and support. We have talked about this, but perhaps it's a pipedream given that we all have very different financial and family circumstances.

There are also some intergenerational co-living models. In the Netherlands, changes to care home standards meant that some rooms no longer met the space requirements for an elderly resident. These spare rooms were let out to students, initially as a way of generating some revenue. In exchange for a discounted rent the students were also asked to give around 30 hours of their time per month to care for their co-residents. I met some of these students on a visit to the Netherlands. One, Arthur, had got to know one of his neighbours and they had become friends. He took him out to the pub to socialise and in return got advice on setting up his own business. The wider benefits of intergenerational living for both students and older residents alike mean the idea is being taken up in the UK and other countries and is being designed into new developments. Novel living arrangements, as well as innovation in home design, could transform how we live in later life, opening up opportunities to remain active and independent, and with greater opportunities for socialising.

The truth is that house building has not kept pace with growing demand. This has fuelled rising house prices and concentrated home ownership in the hands of fewer people, limiting the opportunity to own a home to those whose families already own property. This is society's problem, not one to be blamed on the older generation. The number of older households is set to increase rapidly in the next 20 years, and yet the focus of policy and house builders, in part because of government incentives, is on first-time buyers and family homes.

We must shift the debate from downsizing to right-sizing – recognising the need for a diversity of sizes across tenures, at affordable prices, in the locations where people want to live. We must build all new homes to higher accessibility standards, so that they are able to adapt to the changing needs of the population. If we fail to build new homes that are accessible and adaptable, we will create another housing crisis – rather than the one we see today that is driven by a lack of quantity, we will create one in the future caused by a lack of quality. It is critical that we build more new homes, but it is equally important that we build them 'right'.

And yet the vast majority of homes we will live in for the foreseeable future are already built, so we must also tackle the state of existing housing. The age and condition of much of the housing in the UK means the vast majority of homes are unfit for us as we age. There are lots of things that can and need to be done to overhaul these homes to make them fit for the future. We need to undertake a major retrofit of existing housing to make it warm, safe and adaptable.

The rapid growth in the private rental sector means that in future there will be many more older renters. Stronger regulation of landlords and better rights for tenants would give young and old alike the security they desire. If the private sector can't deliver this, there will need to be additional provision in the social rented sector.

There is a huge opportunity to transform our housing, not only to design homes that are accessible, but also homes that harness technology to enable us to live independently for longer. If we fail to do so, the current housing crisis will only worsen, but we must not forget the social aspects of where we live and who we live with. We turn in the next chapter to the importance of communities to our wellbeing in later life and how the age shift is changing the face of where we live.

9

The loneliness myth and why the place we live matters

'Young or old, loneliness doesn't discriminate.'
Jo Cox, former Labour MP for Batley and Spen

Loneliness has been portrayed as being as bad for your health as smoking 15 cigarettes a day. We are fed images of lonely old people to pull at our heartstrings so we'll donate to charity. And many charities for older people and community organisations see loneliness as a major problem to be tackled. But does it affect older people more than young people? I will challenge the myth that loneliness is a problem of the old and look at who is lonely and why. Most of us have a wide range of social connections, including every-day contact with people in local shops, with neighbours and colleagues. Wider networks of people who can provide support and help when we need it are important, too, particularly when our circumstances change, for example, if we fall ill. But can these relationships really substitute, in emotional terms, for the personal and trusted relationships we have with close friends, a partner or spouse? I'll look at the different kinds of personal and social relationships we need as we age.

Many of the interventions to 'treat' loneliness involve identifying lonely individuals and trying to get them engaged in community activities by 'prescribing' social activity. Does this medicalised approach to curing the 'epidemic of loneliness' work? I will look at the evidence and suggest alternative approaches that focus more on life events and people's ability to build and maintain social networks.

We're seeing significant changes in the way we live. More people are living alone, divorce rates are increasing rapidly at older ages and we are increasingly communicating virtually rather than face to face. Society is becoming more fragmented and there is a worry about the future of our communities. Many activities and spaces are age-segregated, and some think this will further divide the generations. Together with the age shift, what will these changes in the way we live together mean for our later lives? How can we create communities that are inclusive of everyone, of all ages and abilities?

WHO IS LONELY?

Loneliness has been defined as a feeling that arises when there is a gap between the quantity and quality of the social relationships you want and those you have. Loneliness can be a transitory feeling, but when you experience it all or most of the time it is chronic. It is possible to feel lonely even if you have social contact. Perhaps you live with someone, you have a job, you are surrounded by people, but you still feel lonely because you are in an unhappy relationship, you don't get on with your colleagues, or don't know any of your neighbours.

If I asked you to think of someone who was lonely, who comes to mind? Most likely an older person perhaps too disabled or frail to go out, no family nearby and living on their own, having outlived their spouse or partner and many of their friends. Such stereotypes are perhaps not surprising. John Lewis in 2015 partnered with Age UK to run a Christmas TV ad campaign featuring 'the man on the moon'. The charity sought to highlight the million older people in the UK who spend Christmas alone and who can go a month without speaking to a friend, neighbour or family member. The advert generated strong emotions and was guaranteed to make you reach for your wallet or phone to make a donation.

But the impression, bolstered by fundraising ads and other stereotypes, that this kind of sad isolation is the preserve of older people is simply wrong. In fact, the Community Life Survey, funded by the government, which gathers views from more than 10,000 people, mostly online, shows 16- to 24-year-olds are most affected by loneliness. While nearly a third (30%) of 16- to 24-year-olds feel lonely often or sometimes, only 17% of those aged 75 and over said the same thing, with 60% of over 75s reporting that they never or hardly ever felt lonely.[1]

There's a lot more to the issue than simply whether we feel lonely. The quantity and quality of our social relationships matter, too. Social isolation, a concept closely related to loneliness, is usually defined by the number of contacts you have in a defined period of time but having social contact doesn't tell us much about the quality of those relationships. Experts believe that quantity matters more for young people – they expect to have a large social network – whereas as we get older the quality of relationships matters more, for example, having those key confidantes and an inner network.

Another related issue is whether we feel we belong to our community. The same survey mentioned above includes a range of questions which shed light on our social networks and how these are changing. One of the questions is: do you feel you belong to your community? In answer, older people generally report positively – more than two-thirds of over 75s say they feel fairly strongly or strongly that they belong to their neighbourhood, compared to only 40% of 16- to 24-year-olds. And the overwhelming majority (95%+) say they would have someone to rely on in a crisis and there is generally no difference by age. So this seems to paint a more positive picture than the caricature of a lonely old person sitting in front of the TV for companionship. Just because you're old doesn't mean you're lonely, but there's a significant minority who have a tough time and lack social connection. Let's look at the reasons why.

WHY ARE SOME PEOPLE LONELY?

People face many barriers to building and maintaining social contact. These could include a home that is too messy or cold to want to invite people round, or ill health or a disability that makes it hard to get out and about. Such constraints are not just experienced by older people. Parents of young children might find it hard to maintain friendships or refugees might struggle to build social connections without a common language. Across the life course, a number of transitions or life events have been identified that are more commonly associated with loneliness. Moving home, changing schools, seeking asylum, leaving the armed forces, developing a health condition, leaving care, becoming a carer, becoming a parent, changing jobs or leaving work, experiencing family breakdown and bereavement are all potential triggers for loneliness.[2]

In the Later Life Study over 90% of people over the age of 50 reported that they have a friend or family member they can rely on if they have a serious problem, and yet among the 'struggling and alone' group (approximately 12% of the population over 50 across all ages) this fell to 70%. And while over 95% of the thriving baby boomers, who were the happiest group, said they hardly ever or never lacked companionship, as few as one in four of the 'struggling and alone' said the same. Those with long-standing health conditions in the 'struggling and alone' group recognised that their health impacts on their ability to plan social engagements for fear they will not be well enough to participate. They also rely more on people coming to them to visit and over time this results in them becoming more isolated.

Looking across a range of studies, we find that people who experience loneliness and social isolation are more likely to have health conditions, live in poverty or lack money, be out of work or have caring responsibilities. Analysis of one wave of data from the English Longitudinal Study of Ageing categorised people over 50 into six groups. The researchers used sophisticated statistical analysis to cluster people together based on whether their answers to questions about loneliness, social isolation and living alone were similar. Having constructed these groups, they then went on to compare them in terms of the sorts of people in them. The group that experienced no issues with loneliness or social isolation were on average the best educated, while the group with high levels of loneliness, moderate isolation and a high likelihood of living alone had the highest proportion of people from the poorest fifth of the population, as well as the highest proportion of people who were unemployed.[3]

Public Health England has also taken an interest in social isolation. It commissioned the Institute of Health Equity at University College London to look at the evidence on what can be done to reduce social isolation across the life course. The findings confirmed the results of the studies mentioned above: some risk factors are more common in socially disadvantaged groups, including unemployment and illness in later life. These influences accumulate throughout life so isolation at older ages may have roots earlier in life and, as mentioned, other events, such as bereavement, developing a health condition or having caring responsibilities, all reduce social contact.[4] These are more common at older ages and if you already have weaker social networks, this could contribute to social isolation.

We also know that lack of money, poor health and caring responsibilities can be barriers to participation in social activities. While 9 out of 10 older adults aged 50-74 go out socially, those who don't say the things that stop them include poor health and disability, financial reasons, caring responsibilities or not having anyone to go out with. A quarter (24%) of 55- to 59-year-olds who don't go out socially cite financial reasons and one in ten 50- to 59-year-olds talk about the limitations of their caring responsibilities.[5]

The Centre for Ageing Better's review of inequalities found that more older people from BAME backgrounds reported feeling lonely than in the wider population and there is some evidence suggesting that older LGBT+ people are more likely to be socially isolated. People with restrictive health conditions or disabilities, particularly those with reduced mobility, or sight or hearing loss, also report higher levels of loneliness.[6]

While our basic human need for meaningful and personal relationships is a constant and doesn't change as we age, experience and life events across the life course do make some people more likely to be lonely or socially isolated. Let's look at the types of relationships we value and the impact of not having these.

WHAT TYPES OF RELATIONSHIPS MATTER?

Friends are important. They support us through the good times and the bad. They can introduce us to new activities and hobbies when we retire to enable us to develop a new structure and purpose away from work. If we lose our partner, they provide important practical and emotional support. It appears that women are more likely to place a higher value on friendships and invest more time in cultivating them than men. Two-thirds of women over 50 in the Later Life Study said relationships with other people are very important, compared to 56% of men.

But it's clear from the same study that time for making and nurturing friendships is being squeezed for those in mid-life by the pressures of work and caring. The squeezed middle-aged group, also sometimes called the Sandwich Generation, are not investing in friendships, because they are juggling long working hours and family commitments, both to support children and elderly relatives. They are more likely to enter later life with a weaker social support network than some of the people who went before them. And as more women work, on retirement they may face similar challenges to some men, whose social networks are dominated by people they know through work. This is why employers need to support people to plan and prepare for the social and emotional aspects of retirement.

Another challenge as people get older is that friendships can become more difficult to sustain. Health problems may limit our ability to travel or go out and meet friends, or deterioration in hearing can make it hard to join in in a group setting or noisy public place such as a café. Even using the phone as a means of communication can be difficult. There's also a risk that if all our friends are our own age, we'll outlive them or find it more difficult to stay in touch and communicate. My mum, who is in her late 70s, was invited to join a book group made up mostly of professional women in their 50s. She was unsure about joining, thinking she was 'too old'. Despite these doubts, she joined and she now has a group of friends some 20 years younger than her. This both keeps her outlook young and has strengthened her social network, making it more resilient.

Family matters, too, although as more people are living longer and having fewer children, families are becoming 'tall and thin'. In other words, it's becoming more common to have four-generation families with fewer people in each generation. This has implications for the extent of social support and interaction we can expect with our families.

On the upside, it increases the opportunities for inter-generational relationships within families. Those who are grandparents provide a significant amount of childcare, with the value of childcare given by those over 65 estimated to be worth £7.7 billion.[7] There are positive benefits of such contact. For some people we spoke to in the Later Life Study, having provided childcare to their grandchildren, they would feel more able to ask for help if they needed it. Many older people valued this contact as it exposed them to different views. They could learn from younger generations, but also pass on their skills and experience. This, in turn, made people feel valued. One person told us, 'This is the time when my family can say I've got my grandad – my grandad taught me this.'

But on the downside, smaller families means that there are fewer children who can be called upon to provide care and support if needed. If we don't have children, who will be there to look after us and advocate on our behalf when we are too ill or lack the capacity to do this for ourselves?

For the increasing number of people without children there are particular challenges and issues in looking ahead to our old age. Who will be there to support us when we're ill or finding it hard to manage? Who will attend important medical appointments with us? Who will visit us in hospital and make sure that our care is co-ordinated? Who will be there when we are ready to return home? Who will act on our behalf to manage our finances or make informed decisions if we are no longer able to, for example, because of dementia? Who will inherit any wealth we have? Who will arrange the funeral, clear the house and sort out our estate when we die? For those with children, the default answer to most of these questions is their son or daughter. For those with no children, those who are estranged from their children or with kids on the other side of the world, alternative arrangements will have to be made.

Ageing Well Without Children is an organisation that seeks to advocate on behalf of people who don't have children as well as supporting them to plan and prepare for later life. It conducted research with people in this situation and identified that dementia was a particular worry, along with other conditions that would result in people being unable to advocate on their own behalf.[8] Often this worry was triggered when people found themselves caring for their own parents and realised that they might not have the same support when they needed it. I, for one, am investing in relationships with my nieces and nephews. This is not a cynical move(!). I enjoy spending time with them, but I am also now aware that those relationships could be really important to me one day.

While having contact with family can be positive, fewer of us will be able to rely on our children to support us if we need care and support in old age. This decline in the availability of unpaid family care has huge implications for health and care services, as we saw in chapters 6 and 7.

Interviews of people over 50 for our Later Life study asked people about their relationships with family and friends and found that those who were married or living with a partner were less likely to feel they lacked companionship compared to those who were single, divorced or widowed. One person told us, 'No, I don't lack companionship at all because I've got such close family, but it must be awful for people who don't. Having a partner is the most important thing.'

Since I was given the 'Happy to Chat' badge at the launch of the Jo Cox Commission on Loneliness, I have tried to make an effort to stop and chat to the people I pass regularly in my street. People like Peter who has health problems and lives alone. Every morning when I open my curtains he is sitting on the bench in the park opposite my house. When I pass on my way to the swimming pool or work, we say hello and ask each other how we are. He is always happy to chat. I did an impromptu 'interview' with him for this book on my way back from the swimming pool. When I mentioned I was writing a chapter on loneliness, he said he sometimes feels lonely. I asked him why, and he simply said, 'I don't have anyone to talk to.' He went on to say that life was difficult because he feels has to face everything alone. He really wants to find a soulmate, someone he can share everything with, who has no agenda. Peter attends the local Methodist Church and said that his faith makes a difference: 'I feel less alone with God. Going to church keeps me going.'

Whatever other relationships we have, having a significant other has a huge impact on whether we feel lonely or not. Perhaps it is therefore not surprising that dating sites for the over 50s have taken off and *Saga Magazine* has recently launched a new dating column.

As we have seen, there is a wide range of types of social relationships that matter. Many of us will be happy most of the time with the quantity and quality of the relationships we have, but what about those people who experience chronic loneliness, who, for one reason or another, don't have the social relationships that they want or need? What approaches are being taken to address their loneliness?

WHAT IS BEING DONE TO ADDRESS LONELINESS?

The focus of policy, as well as many interventions, is on tackling loneliness by targeting individuals who are *already* experiencing loneliness. One of the challenges with these models is that people who are lonely often find it hard to reach out for help. One way of identifying people is through their GP.

Social prescribing has become quite widespread in the NHS among GPs as a means of signposting people who could benefit from accessing social and community activities. Dr Zoe Wyrko, who I mentioned in a previous chapter, is sceptical about this approach. She says, 'Why are we introducing the word "prescribing" to something that is actually just about living?' Many of these people will have health issues – part of the reason they are lonely in the first place – and will need more than signposting to re-engage in social activities. For example, they might have lost their confidence and need someone to accompany them, or practical support, to overcome the barriers which have prevented them from going out. For some people, it may be long-standing mental health issues that are the underlying reason and, unless these are recognised and treated, other efforts to get them along to groups will likely fail.

The NHS Long Term Plan has signalled it will fund community link workers. While there hasn't been much detail yet on what they will do, it is likely they will build on the experience of the National Lottery Community Fund programmes around the country, which included roles like 'community connectors', who helped to facilitate engagement and support people who were socially isolated or feeling lonely into activities that suit them. A similar model, called Living Well, was implemented in Cornwall, in partnership with Age UK (see box opposite).

LIVING WELL IN CORNWALL

Living Well is a scheme launched in 2012 that brings together local health, statutory and community services to provide 'wrap-around' care to better support people with long-term conditions at risk of hospital admission. The aim is to build resilience and a stronger support network for those at risk of social isolation or loneliness. The schemes set out to support the person in their community and help them to meet their goals, such as being able to walk for longer stretches of time or connect with new people. Initial findings suggest that these joined up services have reduced GP appointments, hospital admissions and have saved the local authority money.[9]

This approach risks medicalising the problem and by 'prescribing' social activities as the remedy fails to address some of the more fundamental causes. Although loneliness is associated with poor health, it is not a 'disease' to be treated with a prescription in the same way that doctors might treat diabetes or heart failure. Dr Kalpa Kharicha, Head of Innovation, Policy and Research at the Campaign to End Loneliness, argues that the national conversation on loneliness needs to change: 'I think it's important to differentiate between transient and chronic loneliness and recognise loneliness is a normal emotion experienced by many people; it shouldn't be turned into an "epidemic". The language of loneliness needs to be used responsibly, and I think shouldn't promote ageist stereotypes about vulnerability and older people being a drain on services.'

A range of interventions have been tried to address loneliness over recent years. The majority of these have been aimed at older adults. They include group and individual interventions, some delivered face to face and others through digital means. All sorts of leisure activities, including gardening, music and physical activity, have been tried, as well as more focused education and training programmes. According to a recent review, while many did not have any effect, those that taught self-management approaches that included practising social skills were successful.[10]

Befriending and social and community interventions are very common, and a huge amount of voluntary and community sector activity goes into helping people, either one to one or in groups, to re-engage in local activities and networks. Open Age, which is a charity operating across the London boroughs of Kensington and Chelsea, Westminster and Hammersmith and Fulham, has a buddy system. If someone is identified as being chronically lonely or has lost confidence, the buddy will visit them at their home (rather than simply befriending them), will get to know more about them and their interests, and gradually encourage them to try out one of the many activities offered by Open Age. The buddy will also accompany them for the first few times to ensure they get settled into the group.

It is not clear whether these interventions work to reduce loneliness. The same review identified some promising research to suggest that advice, signposting or community-based programmes designed to build confidence and encourage networking do reduce loneliness, but there have only been a few research studies with small numbers of participants, which makes it difficult to say whether any interventions of the type I mention above work.

As we have seen, there are things that make us more likely to become lonely or socially isolated and certain transitions may weaken our social contacts. A life-course approach, which targets people during transitions that we know people find problematic, such as bereavement, diagnosis of a new health condition or suddenly needing to care for others, might therefore be more effective. Other interventions could also be useful, including pre-retirement courses that help people with the emotional and psychological aspects of retirement, and social opportunities for those who are separated, divorced or widowed. Findings from less rigorous and non-academic studies have generally indicated that personalised support at trigger points would be useful, but there has been no pilot or wide-scale study of this. Late Spring is a great example of a scheme that supports recently bereaved people (see box below).

LATE SPRING – HELPING BEREAVED PEOPLE RE-CONNECT

Late Spring is a network of bereavement support groups in Oxfordshire that gives people over 60 who have recently lost a loved one the opportunity to meet over coffee and cake. While these are not counselling sessions, talking about the loss is encouraged, as is looking towards the future. There are specific groups for specific communities, both geographic and social, who meet on a regular basis.

Robert, a widower who served in the RAF for 35 years, found the support invaluable: 'I wanted to meet people that were in a similar situation, because, as I said, you can't talk to your own family and friends about stuff like that. You can, but you can't keep doing that. But when you go to Late Spring you can keep talking about it and it's a warm feeling to be quite honest, because you are talking to these people and you're keeping your memories, not just in your head, you're actually bringing them out into the open so they're shared by the people. I think that's a wonderful thing to be quite honest.'

Interventions which focus on life transitions and provide support at the moments when people most need it are promising and should be evaluated to find out if they make a difference to whether people feel lonely and the extent of their social connections. However, if we want to take a more preventative approach, we need to do more at a community level to create the conditions for social connections to thrive. Let's look at how existing community provision is trying to make a difference to older people's social connections and how this might need to change.

COMMUNITY ACTIVITIES

Most of the current community provision run by the voluntary and community sector provides social activities for older people. I recently visited Armley Helping Hands in Leeds. It's based in a community centre in quite a deprived neighbourhood and provides a wide range of community activities. The day I visited I met Jim, who was playing dominoes with his friend in a reminiscence room decorated with photos and furniture typical of a home of the 1950s. When Jim retired, he felt that this sort of activity was not for him. He didn't see himself as old, but recently he had been in touch with his local MP who had encouraged him to attend a supper club that they were running. This was just the encouragement he needed. He enjoyed the evening so much he has been coming back regularly, taking part in activities up to three days a week. Jim has no family and lost touch many years ago with his brother, so had very little social contact before coming to Armley Helping Hands.

Jim is collected from his home by community buses owned and run by the organisation. Talking to Dawn, who runs the organisation, it's clear that providing transport is vital to enable local residents to get out and attend social activities, but community transport is expensive to run and the organisation spends a lot of time and effort fundraising to keep it going. It also arranges transport to take people to hospital, doctor's appointments and the shops. I met one of the drivers, Denis, who had previously been a long-distance lorry driver. He clearly enjoyed meeting the older residents he picked up and dropped off and got to know them well. If he had any concerns about any of those he was regularly picking up, he was able to get help from other local services.

In my view the benefits of small neighbourhood organisations like Armley Helping Hands are less about whether someone attends a bingo club or a supper club or a dance, and much more about the staff and volunteers at the centre who care about the people who come, look out for them if they don't seem so good, and make sure they are managing OK at home. The Centre for Ageing Better is evaluating schemes like this across Leeds to understand more systematically whether and how they impact on the health and wellbeing of older residents, as well as on the use of NHS services. It is this vital network of support that is missing in so many neighbourhoods and particularly for people who don't have family. Dawn was clear that even if there is family, they are not always able to help. They have their own challenges and difficulties, and relationships are not always that easy. Services need to do a much better job of harnessing the good will of communities and volunteers by building a relationship with people in their neighbourhood who can keep an eye out and support people before they hit crisis, and thus avert more expensive care.

But schemes like Armley Helping Hands struggle to attract people who do not identify themselves as old or in need (other than as volunteers). Dr Kalpa Kharicha, the expert from Campaign to End Loneliness I spoke to earlier, reminded me, 'You'll want to continue doing things you enjoy doing and you've done all your life, so helping people maintain those interests is really important. Nobody wants to go to a club for lonely old people. That's the crux of it.' A challenge is how to make community activities more inclusive and appealing to a wide range of people. This will mean engaging people in an activity or social event based around an interest, hobby or place, rather than age. For example, we might come together with others with whom we share religious beliefs or cultural heritage or to improve the place we live, either through formal tenants' associations or a clean-up of the local park.

Many community activities and some facilities are age-segregated – think about schools, day centres, old people's homes, nightclubs. Does contact with other generations matter? Age segregation in communities more generally can lead to a paucity of social contact across generations. Elaine, Chair of Greater Manchester's Older People Network, a group set up to inform and influence policies affecting older people in Greater Manchester, talked about the need for inclusive communities. 'As you get older you still want to stay in your community – and "community" does not just mean older people together, it means younger people, middle-aged people, where you mix together.'

There are high-profile examples of how generations are coming together, with care homes now co-locating with children's nurseries and students renting rooms in older people's residential homes, something which started in the Netherlands, but has caught on elsewhere as we saw in the chapter on housing. In the US, many thousands of older volunteers are involved in Experience Corps. They go into schools to help young people with their reading, in particular. Evaluation of this found that not only did the children's educational outcomes improve, but the older people also benefitted from the contact.[11] Similar schemes operate in schools in the UK, but not on the same scale as across the US. Leading gerontologist, Professor Christina Victor, was wary of the possible tokenism of this. 'We might want to think a bit more creatively about intergenerational social engagement,' she said, 'and I don't just mean taking a few primary school kids into a care home. We definitely should resist going down the route of gated communities where you're forced to live with people your own age. Perhaps it's about how we plan our cities and environment, so people of different ages interact.'

If you want to live a long and happy life, you might want to move to one of the so-called 'blue zones', places in the world where there are a very high proportion of centenarians, for example, the island of Okinawa in Japan, where the proportion of centenarians is 24.55 for every 100,000 inhabitants. They live by the principle of *ichariba chode*, which means 'Treat everyone like a brother, even if you've never met them before.'[12] The secret to their happiness is that they feel part of a community and help each other out. The residents are part of a *moai* – an informal group of people with common interests who look out for each other. People contribute financially to support the activities of the group and funds can be used to provide financial support to a member of the group who finds themselves in financial difficulty. It is often the social aspects of community life as much as the physical infrastructure that determines whether older people feel able to participate in their community. Could the UK declare one of our cities or regions a blue zone and try to replicate the extraordinary success of these long-living communities?

Even if we could create different opportunities for people of all ages to engage in community activities, if we are to take a preventative approach, we need to hardwire social connections into the fabric of our communities.

CREATING COMMUNITY

Much of our day-to-day social interaction happens in the places we live and work. Where we live makes a difference to our ability to build social networks. How does the design of places influence whether we are connected with our neighbours, whether we are able to get out and about, and whether we feel we belong?

Professor Victor has also suggested that our built environment is not designed to facilitate social interaction: 'The structure of our environment is such that you can't get to the library to go to the community class because there isn't a bus or you have to cross an eight-lane highway, so getting policy makers to think about the physical infrastructure is important, and creating places where people can meet.'

There are several league tables rating how friendly towns and cities across the UK are. In general, older people are happy with the place they live. Data from the Community Life Survey found that people aged 65 and over were more likely to be satisfied with their local area compared to younger age groups (84% compared to 75% of those aged 25-34). By far the biggest factor in people's satisfaction with their local area relates to its level of deprivation, with just 60% of people living in the most deprived areas satisfied with where they live compared with 88% in the least deprived areas.[13]

Austerity has certainly had an impact on communities. The same survey found that the proportion of people who say their area has got worse in the last two years has gone up from 20% in

2013-2014 to 24% in 2017-2018. Cuts to local authority budgets have resulted in closures of libraries and community centres, reducing public spaces where it is (usually) free for people to go and which provide low-cost facilities for community groups to meet. As well as the impact of austerity, the decline of the high street is also seen as a factor in losing a sense of community. As internet shopping reduces the footfall and spend on the high street, shops are closing and becoming concentrated in larger urban centres, which can attract more high value shoppers. If everything moves online, what happens to those small social interactions we used to have in the Post Office, the bank and at the supermarket? There is a risk that our neighbourhoods will feel unsafe, unfriendly and uninviting for older and younger people alike. The consequences are less money going into the local economy, fewer local jobs and a spiral of decline.

Local authorities and businesses need to come together to find new solutions for the high street. Some councils are being innovative and looking at how to make use of other community facilities, opening up spaces in leisure centres, in GP surgeries and children's centres to other users. We need places like schools and village halls, as well as pubs and cafés, to be spaces where people of all ages can meet and interact. We also need to focus on investing in deprived communities – these are the areas where it's harder for communities to flourish. There are fewer amenities and green spaces. Community businesses can potentially play a role in ensuring some amenities remain on local high streets.

Recently, my husband was walking along the high street in the town he grew up in. Looking around he realised there were hardly any places he recognised – the library was long gone, many local shops closed, replaced by betting shops and fast food outlets, the big old pubs pulled down and redeveloped as flats. Only the church and the police station were still recognisable, although the latter was under wraps, being redeveloped into housing. My mother-in-law, who lived there, didn't feel safe going down the high street and there was little reason to. She had to be driven to a bank in another town as she didn't trust online banking.

We need a radical revisioning of the high street to create a place where people of all ages and incomes want to come and meet and play. It means having streets that are safe and walkable – easy to manage for people who move more slowly or have mobility difficulties. There may be fewer shops, but this could create an opportunity for more residential spaces.

The Conservative government in 2019 made £675 million of funding available to support local authorities to develop proposals for the regeneration of 'struggling town centres' where the turnover of shops is high. Some of the retail space is being converted to housing, but unfortunately permitted development means that converted properties do not need to meet housing standards which otherwise apply to new buildings. This means they are often small and do not meet accessibility requirements or even the basics everyone would assume. A housing developer is currently trying to convert ex-industrial space in Watford into residential units – with no windows! If retail space is converted into housing, planners must be given the powers to ensure these meet local need, with accessible housing and other essential services and amenities, such as GP practices, required as part of the redevelopment. Encouraging older people to 'right-size' into accessible developments in or near town centres could be just the thing to create vibrant all-age communities.

There are some innovations that are trying to buck the trend. Chatty cafés have sprung up and even big supermarkets like Sainsburys are getting on board by having one larger table in the café where people are encouraged to sit and chat to each other. Since its launch in 2017, more than a thousand cafes have signed up to the scheme and designated a 'chatter and natter' table to facilitate conversation. This initiative was awarded an Innovating for Ageing award by the International Longevity Centre, a think-tank dedicated to the impact of longevity in 2019.

For bigger retailers, too, finding ways of reaching older people who are less digitally connected could seriously boost profits, while making a real difference to the lives of people who have become increasingly locked out of using the shops and services they want. One innovative solution is the 'high street showroom', where people can view products before ordering them in store. This can help bridge the digital divide for people without access to, or are uncomfortable with, online shopping, while allowing retailers to retain the cost-efficiency of large out-of-town warehouses.

Having access to green space means we are more active and also creates opportunities to meet other people, when we're out walking the dog, running or just sitting on a park bench. And yet again, maintenance of green spaces falls to councils who, when facing tighter budgets, often cut back on these 'non-essential' services. If parks don't look or feel safe, fewer people will use them. Deprived areas are more likely to lack both adequate public spaces and green spaces, which can create barriers to social interaction. Creating places where social connections flourish requires local authorities, citizens, housing developers, public services and businesses to work together and reimagine communities. Some places are already beginning to do this.

WHAT IS AN AGE-FRIENDLY COMMUNITY?

A growing number of forward-thinking cities and communities around the world are committed to becoming age-friendly, but what is an age-friendly city or community? According to Andrew Cuomo, Governor of New York state, which was designated the first age-friendly state in the US by the World Health Organisation in 2017, it's about 'designing communities for everyone that strengthen people's connections to each other, improve health, increase physical activity and support, and advance the economic environment through proactive design and future-based planning.'[14] It involves understanding the needs of older residents and engaging them in developing plans, such as transport strategy, infrastructure planning and defining the housing needs of the future. Planners and designers need to consider how older residents use spaces, and the journeys and routes they take. The design of housing and transport needs to be inclusive and accessible to enable people of all ages and abilities to get out and about.

The World Health Organisation brought together 33 cities from 22 countries in 2006 to consider how the urban environment needed to change to support active and healthy ageing. The World Health Organisation's Age-Friendly Communities Framework, which resulted from this, is made up of eight 'domains' that cover both the social and built environment: outdoor spaces and buildings, transport, housing, social participation, respect and social inclusion, civic participation and employment, communication and information, and community support and health services. There were 760 age-friendly communities and cities worldwide in 2018 and the movement is growing all the time. Manchester was the first UK city to sign up to the Age-Friendly Communities Framework in 2010 and there were 34 age-friendly communities across the UK in 2019.

The approach engages older people in the process and looks across all the policies and services which shape a place. Practical changes can involve schemes like Take a Seat, which encourages local businesses to provide a seat for anyone who might need one, with no obligation to buy. Another campaign, called Caught Short, advocated for more public toilets, and for shops and businesses not to restrict the use of toilets to customers. In the Isle of Wight, the local bus company gave training to all its drivers so that they better understood the different needs of older customers. They also issued simple cards to customers, for example, with sight impairment or mobility difficulties, to show to the driver so they knew to call out the stop or wait until passengers were seated before pulling off. Other innovations include cards which can be swiped at pedestrian crossings to allow extra crossing time.

The design of the built environment is critical to enable people to continue to remain active and connected. On one estate in Greater Manchester, called Old Moat, the housing association engaged residents in redesigning the estate to make it more age-friendly. This included straightforward things like more benches and places for people to sit down, but also raised redirecting bus routes so it was easier to reach the health centre and hospital without changing buses.

Public transport is vital to enable people to get out and about. The lack of transport in rural areas means that people are much more likely to become socially isolated. If only one bus per week runs into the local town, it is little use if you can't carry a week's shopping, or if the doctor's appointment you need to attend happens to be on a different day to the one the bus runs on, or the activity you want to do is in the evening after the bus has stopped running. It is important that new modes of transport are tested with older people and those in rural areas and that new approaches including using technology to recruit and manage volunteer drivers, as well as making more efficient use of community transport, are developed.[15]

When people need or want to stop driving in later life due, for example, to loss of sight or other impairments caused by health issues, this has an obvious impact on their ability to take part in social activities. Lack of confidence using public transport or reluctance to use taxis means that, even where these are available, older people may leave their homes less frequently when they give up driving. I met a friend of my mum's recently who has macular degeneration, a gradual deterioration in sight which mainly affects older people. She had begun to look at options to move nearer to the town centre as they currently relied on the car. But then her son-in-law worked out that they could take two or three taxis a day for the rest of their lives for the same amount it was going to cost them to move. The estate agent who had come to value the house that same week agreed. For her, using taxis was a better solution than moving from a house that they were happy in and suited them in every other way.

Driving cessation is a problem, so could driverless cars be the answer? Let's look at whether technology could transform our social lives.

THE FUTURE

There is growing interest in harnessing smart technologies to keep people connected and promote social contact, and physical and mental wellbeing. Affordable access to driverless cars could enable older people who find it difficult to use public transport or don't have access to it, but there are some very practical challenges to extending them to rural areas where public transport is most likely to be limited and the need for people in later life is greatest.

The way we communicate is rapidly changing. Younger generations are not making phone calls any more, with less than two-thirds of smartphone owners (69%) making a phone call within the last week in 2016, compared to nearly all (96%) in 2012.[16] Communication is now real time through social media channels that have the ability to send images, text, and recorded voice and video messages instantaneously. Everywhere you look there are people with their heads down looking at their phones or with headphones in. They are 'connected', but not to the people around them and the contact is not face to face.

As society becomes ever more automated and digitised, as self-checkouts and online banking become ever more prevalent, as advice bots replace the people at call centres, will we have less human contact? Home delivery by drones might even mean the end to the friendly chat with the home delivery driver. But is social contact through a digital interface different in quality from face-to-face social contact? We don't know yet how this will impact on social relationships or how we feel. There is some evidence to link use of social media with loneliness and mental health problems in young people.[17] If we don't have the skills or experience of making deeper personal relationships early in life, there is the potential that we will be at a greater risk of social isolation in later life, but there is also some research showing that older people who were taught video conferencing so they could communicate with family who did not live close by were less lonely.[18]

Could virtual communities replace real communities where people meet because of a common interest or shared hobby? Even if we became housebound, we could interact with our grandchildren on the other side of the world at the touch of a screen or participate in online book groups or discussion forums. In fact, whatever our interest we could connect in virtual communities to other people who share that interest. The use of virtual reality, for example, could be used to enable someone who is otherwise housebound to explore places like museums and galleries with friends.

One of the things that struck me at the New Old exhibition I went to at London's Design Museum was how some technologies that are already available could be harnessed to make life so much easier for someone with mobility or other challenges. The voice-activated system linked to a computer called ElliQ could enable someone who is not digitally skilled to interact with friends, family and online services more intuitively. The computer can ask whether you want to see some photos your granddaughter has just sent you or hear a message from the local library. The widespread adoption of voice-activated products will rapidly transform how we access digital services and may overcome some of the barriers some people in later life have faced in using them. And yet older people are less likely to be online or have a smartphone and digital exclusion is a barrier to staying connected with friends and family, accessing local transport and participating in community activities.[19]

Loneliness is not a 'disease of old age' to be feared, but something that can happen at any life stage, so the age shift in our society doesn't necessarily mean an epidemic of loneliness. Currently people in later life are generally faring OK when it comes to relationships and feeling part of their community. However, there are some life events and circumstances which leave some of us without the social support and relationships we need as we age. Those who are poor, have ill health or a disability or caring responsibilities are all at higher risk of experiencing loneliness and social isolation. Bereavement, divorce or losing a job are all triggers for loneliness, too. While it may seem like many of these are very personal experiences over which society as a whole has very little influence, mitigating the impact of these changes is possible, and more services and interventions need to be developed and tested which support people through these life events.

At an individual level there are many ways in which we can tackle and prevent loneliness. Each and every one of us can let people know we are 'happy to chat'. The stronger our social networks, particularly of close friends, the more resilient we are when these events happen. For some of us at least, relying on family is unlikely to provide the support we need in later life and increasingly we will need to look to wider networks of support in our communities, so we also need to change our society.

Critical to addressing this will be to end the age segregation in our communities and to make them places where people of all ages and abilities are included. It means the design of high streets and transport infrastructure needs to be rethought, and there needs to be a much greater level of investment in communities to maintain places and spaces where people can meet and where community activities for all ages can flourish. While trends in technology and the way we communicate could result in greater fragmentation of our communities and increase social isolation, we face choices about the future. In the final chapter of the book I'll look at how we take steps now to create the age of ageing better.

10

Creating the Age of Ageing Better

The doom-mongers' predictions are that the dramatic age shift in our population will have a catastrophic impact on our society: the costs of the state pension will bankrupt the Exchequer; intergenerational conflict will grow as resentment builds up among working adults having to pay taxes to fund age-related benefits for older people; pressures on health and social care will become unsustainable as services are overwhelmed by rising numbers of frail older people; home ownership will remain out of reach for younger generations while older generations hold onto their over-sized homes worth hundreds of thousands; secure jobs and career progression will become a thing of the past as older workers choose not to retire and hold on to the top jobs; and as more older people live alone there will be an epidemic of loneliness. These are the some of the predictions we hear and there is a risk that we start to believe these as truths, that they become a self-fulfilling prophecy.

We have explored together the extent to which these catastrophic predictions are based in fact. While the age shift has its challenges, the dire consequences are often overstated; the growing numbers of older people are often an easy scapegoat for the consequences of other things, like austerity or a chronic shortage of homes; and the solutions proposed are based on a poor understanding of the drivers and barriers to change. Having got the facts straight, it is clear that there are other solutions: we have choices. And it is not too late. If we act with urgency today, we still have chance to create an age of ageing better. The age shift is only now upon us as the baby boomers of the 1960s enter later life. In this final chapter I set out an alternative future and the actions which can make it a reality.

THE WORLD OF AGEING BETTER

In chapter 2 I invited you to imagine a dystopian world of ageing badly. Now imagine the *world of ageing better* – a utopian future in 2040.

Technology has been harnessed by companies to augment human workers, enabling physically demanding jobs to be done by people of all ages without damaging their health and enhancing mental processing. Productivity has soared, boosting economic growth, and there are more good quality jobs. Since the government introduced a digital sales tax on the global technology giants, public finances have been in the black.

More people are working for longer and paying taxes for longer as well. As a result, the state pension has increased and pensioner poverty is a thing of the past. Many more people with health conditions are supported to work, and the few who can't work get early access to their pension and are supported to volunteer. Everyone has a mid-life MOT at 50 and has a personal lifelong learning account which gives them access to opportunities to reskill and retrain to keep up with the rapidly changing labour market.

Older entrepreneurs have been encouraged to partner with younger entrepreneurs, combining technology know-how and experience, with more start-ups succeeding than ever before. Small- and medium-size businesses are flourishing. The price of oil and climate change has driven consumers to seek out products and services from local suppliers and local markets, and town centres are thriving.

A movement to create age-friendly communities means high streets are busy with people of all ages. A major investment in accessible and clean public transport means it is easy for people of all ages and abilities to get around. A ban on private vehicle ownership in 2030 means everyone has affordable access to driverless cars when they need to. Rural areas are repopulating as they become better connected to services and drones ensure delivery of services to remote areas.

A major government initiative to focus on prevention and healthy ageing 20 years previously means more people are living longer in good health. Government regulations to reduce sugar and a major investment in communities to boost physical activity with active travel options, a network of public transport and green spaces where people of all ages can get out and about and keep active have reversed obesity trends.

A significant house building programme of energy efficient and accessible homes two decades ago means there are lots of options for people in later life to move and remain independent. As a result, there are fewer falls and admissions to hospitals and care homes are dropping.

The world of ageing better need not remain a distant dream. Public policy decisions we take today, actions by government, by employers, by businesses, by public services, by individuals can put us on a path towards the world of ageing better.

If we do nothing, there is a risk that more and more people in later life will experience poverty, ill health and hardship in future decades. There is a risk that the divisions in our society will become entrenched.

TAKING ACTION FOR A BETTER FUTURE

If we are to enjoy the age of ageing better and avoid the age of ageing badly, we need to be prepared to take bold action.

We must wake up to reality. The age shift is upon us and upon us now. These changes in the age profile of the population should not have taken us by surprise. The large birth cohort born in the

1960s has been there largely unchanged, just getting older one year at a time. And yet both the public and private sector have failed to address these issues with the urgency required.

We must tackle the doom-mongers head on. We must combat everyday ageism in the language, advertising and marketing all around us. We must tackle age discrimination and use the powers in the Equality Act to do so. We must be honest about the pressures on public spending and the choices we face about how we raise taxes (who pays and how much), as well as what we spend it on (who gains). We must stop fuelling intergenerational conflict. Making current older generations the bogeymen and bogeywomen for issues like low economic growth, woeful housing supply and the impact of austerity is grossly misleading.

We must build intergenerational consensus on the changes that are needed. This can't be about old versus young. Rather, it's about how we create a society that everyone – regardless of their age, income or background – can enjoy every stage of life. We must find solutions that work for people of all ages and eliminate the inequalities people in every generation face. For example, local authorities' local plans, house designers and developers should consider the needs of both young and old. Government should legislate to introduce secure tenancies which will benefit young and old alike. Employers and government should invest in lifelong training, which would benefit everyone from 16 to 60. Workers of all ages need protections from insecure work.

The whole of national government must commit to take action. It has been internationally recognised that the response to the age shift requires action from every part of government. Angel Gurria, Secretary General of the Organisation of Economic Co-operation and Development (OECD), has written, 'Designing successful policy packages [for healthy ageing] requires rethinking the way policy is made. The evidence on how inequalities compound over the life cycle calls for joint action by ministries and agencies responsible for family, education, health and employment policies at different levels of government.' Countries like Singapore, New Zealand and Australia all have national ageing strategies. The UK must not be left behind globally.

Our response must be cross-sectoral. It requires action from the public, private and community and voluntary sectors; from small local businesses and large national and multi-national corporations; from retail, construction, the digital tech providers and the creative industries; from across the public services, the NHS, local government and Job Centres. Headline-grabbing proposals like abolishing free TV licenses based on age risk distracting from the big structural changes needed across pensions, health, housing and work, as well as changes by individuals, and within families and communities. This does not touch on one part of our lives – it is our lives.

Local leaders must commit to creating age-friendly communities in our cities, towns and villages. Vibrant communities are those which are inclusive of people of all ages. Local authorities must prioritise improving local transport, so it is affordable and accessible, and include the views and voices of people of all ages in the development and redesign of local services.

Industry must be imaginative and come up with new solutions. There are many examples of how innovative products and services could transform later life: new homes that are both green and adaptable; community-based models of care and support that create new forms of 'family' care; new approaches to employment support and volunteering that recognise the skills, experience and assets of the individual; driverless cars to connect people in rural communities to the things they want to do; virtual reality to enable those with limited mobility to remain active and connected to the things they enjoy, and to share the experience with others. New and existing technologies must be harnessed in ways that promote positive ageing and are affordable and accessible to all.

In this book I have set out radical solutions to transform our workplaces, our homes, and our communities, and how we spend our time and use our money. We should see our longer lives as an opportunity. But we must act now to ensure everyone can enjoy their later life. We have the opportunity to create a better future for all of us. The age of ageing better is not a pipe dream, a utopia that is only attainable by the few. It can and must be a reality for the many.

References

INTRODUCING THE AGE OF AGEING BETTER

1 YouGov (2018), poll of 6,943 UK adults over 16, 12-20 February 2018.
2 Abrams, D., Russell, PS, Vauclair, C-M and Swift, H. (2011), *Ageism in Europe: Findings from the European Social Survey*, Age UK.
3 United Nations (2017), Profiles of Ageing.
4 National Institute on Ageing and World Health Organisation (2011), *Global Health and Ageing*.

CHAPTER 1 THE CHANGING FACE OF THE POPULATION

1 Jenkins, J. (2018), 'Preparing for an Aging World', *AARP International: The Journal*, vol. 11- 2018 Edition.
2 Office of National Statistics (2017), Life expectancy at birth and at age 65 by local areas, UK.
3 Office of National Statistics (2017), National Life Tables: UK 2015-2017.
4 Office of National Statistics (2018), Average age at death - by sex, UK.
5 Office of National Statistics (2017), Causes of death over 100 years.
6 Public Health England (2018), *A review of recent trends in mortality in England*.
7 Office of National Statistics (2016), Deaths registered in England and Wales (Series DR): 2015.
8 Office of National Statistics (2018), Deaths registered in England and Wales (series DR): 2006-2017.
9 Department of Health and Social Care (2016), *An Overview of the Death Certificate Reforms*.

10   Office of National Statistics (2018), Deaths registered in England and Wales (series DR), 2006-2017.

11   NHS England, British Medical Association and NHS Employers (2018), *2018/19 General Medical Services (GMS) Contract Quality and Outcomes Framework (QOF)*.

12   Prince, M., Knapp, M., Guerchet, M., McCrone, P., Prina, M., Comas-Herrera, A., Wittenberg, R., Adelaja, B., Hu, B., King, D., Rehill, A. and Salimkumar, D. (2014), *Dementia UK: Second Edition*, Alzheimer's Society.

13   Office of National Statistics (2016), Life expectancy at birth and at age 65 years by local areas, UK, 2011-13 and 2015-17.

14   Public Health England (2018), *A review of recent trends in mortality in England*.

15   Office of National Statistics (2019), Health state life expectancies by Index of Multiple Deprivation (IMD): England, all ages.

16   Raleigh, V. (2018), 'England's stalling life expectancy—pointers for action?', *BMJ Opinion*.

17   Case, A. and Deaton, A. (2017), *Mortality and morbidity in the 21st century*, Brookings Papers on Economic Activity.

18   Zhang, Y., Saito, Y. and Crimmins, E. (2019), 'Changing impact of obesity on active life expectancy of older Americans', *The Journals of Gerontology: Series A* 74:12, pp.1944-1951.

19   Office of National Statistics (2016) Estimates of the very old, including centenarians, UK: mid-2002 to mid-2016 (provisional).

20   United Nations (2017), *World Population Prospects 2017*.

21   Evans, J. (2011), *Differences in life expectancy between those aged 20, 50 and 80 in 2011 and at birth*, Department for Work and Pensions.

22   Gratton, L. and Scott, A. (2016) *The 100-year life: Living and working in an age of longevity*, Bloomsbury: London.

23   Christensen. K., et al. (2009), 'Ageing populations: The challenge ahead', *The Lancet*, 374:9696, pp. 1196–1208.

24   Horn, D. (2018), 'Opinion: The men who want to live forever,' *New York Times*, 27 January 2018.

25   Fries, J.F. (1980), 'Aging, natural death and the compression of morbidity', *New England Journal of Medicine* 303:3, pp. 130–35.

26   O'Dea, C. and Sturrock, D. (2018), *Subjective expectations of survival and economic behaviour*, Institute for Fiscal Studies, Working Paper W18/14.

27 Office of National Statistics (2000), Population estimates – local authority based by five-year age band, mid-year estimates.

28 Office of National Statistics (2018), Estimates of the population for the UK, England and Wales, Scotland and Northern Ireland, mid-2017.

29 Office of National Statistics (2017), table A2-1, Principal projection – UK population in age groups, 2016-based.

30 Office of National Statistics (2018), *How do the post war baby boom generations compare?*

31 Office of National Statistics (2018), Vital statistics in the UK: births, deaths and marriages- 2018 based.

32 Office of National Statistics (2018), Births in England and Wales: summary tables, live births per year, 1960-1969.

33 Cribb, J., Hood, A. and Joyce, R. (2016), *The economic circumstances of different generations: the latest picture*, Institute for Fiscal Studies, Briefing Note BN187.

34 Office of National Statistics (2019), Estimates of the population for the UK, England and Wales, Scotland and Northern Ireland by five-year age group, 1992-2018.

35 United Nations (2017), *Global Profiles of Ageing*.

36 Japanese Ministry of Internal Affairs and Communications (2013), *Housing and Land Survey*.

37 UN Population Division (2017), *Profiles of Ageing: Japan*.

38 Organisation for Economic Co-operation and Development (2014), *Japan: Advancing the third arrow for a resilient economy and inclusive growth*, Better Policy Series.

39 Andrews, K., Minister for Ageing (2001), *National strategy for an ageing Australia: An older Australia, challenges and opportunities for all*, Department of Health.

40 Dalziel, L. (2001), *The New Zealand Positive Ageing Strategy*, Ministry of Social Policy.

41 United Nations (2017), *Profiles of Ageing: UK*.

42 Ministry of Health (2016), *I feel young in my Singapore: Action Plan for Successful Ageing*.

43 Office of National Statistics (2019), table A01: Summary of labour market statistics, July- September 2019.

44 Office of National Statistics, (2018), Household satellite account: full UK accounts 2005 to 2016, table 10, 2016-based estimates.

45 Vass, J., et al. (2014), *Agenda for Later Life 2014: Public Policy for Later Life*, Age UK.
46 United Nations (2017), *Profiles of Ageing: UK.*

CHAPTER 2 WE'RE ALL DOOMED

1 Willetts, D. (2019), *The Pinch: How the baby boomers stole their children's future- and why they should give it back*, 2nd Edition, Atlantic: London, pg. 290.
2 Walker, K. (2011), 'Britain's age timebomb: Cost of 1.4m extra pensioners 'means NHS cannot stay free', *Daily Mail.*
3 Poulter, S. (2012), 'Britain faces old age poverty timebomb as one in five put NOTHING in a pension', *Daily Mail.*
4 Swinford, S. (2013), 'Britain needs millions more immigrants to reduce strain of ageing population', *The Telegraph.*
5 Glaze, B. (2015), 'National debt will hit unsustainable levels by 2060s because of rising elderly population says watchdog', *Daily Mirror.*
6 Williams, A. and Ylanne, V. (2010), 'Portrayals of older adults in UK magazine advertisements: Relevance of target audience', *Communications* 35:1, pp. 1-27.
7 Calouste Gulbenkian and Royal Society for Public Health (2018), *That age old question: How attitudes to ageing affect our health and wellbeing*, Royal Society for Public Health.
8 Ipsos Mori (2014), Perils of perception, survey of 11,527 interviews with people 16-64 in 14 countries.
9 Ipsos Mori (2018), Ipsos Global Advisor, 18,262 adults (16-64) in 29 countries, 24th August-7th September 2018.
10 Centre for Ageing Better (2015), *Later life in 2015: An analysis of the views and experiences of people aged 50 and over*, Ipsos MORI.
11 Swift, H., Abrams, D., Lamont, R. and Drury, L. (2017), 'The risks of ageism model: How ageism and negative attitudes toward age can be a barrier to active ageing', *Social Issues and Policy Review* 11:1 pp. 195-231.
12 Ipsos Global Advisor (2018), Survey of 20,778 adults (16-64) in 30 countries, 24th August-8th September 2018.
13 MHP Health (2014), *Access all ages 2: Exploring variations in access to surgery among older people*, Age UK and Royal College of Surgeons.

14 Centre for Ageing Better (2018), Age discrimination in the workplace, survey of 4,064 GB adults over 50, 19 July-3 August 2018, Ipsos Mori.

15 Levy, B. and Myers, L.M. (2004), 'Preventive health behaviours influenced by self-perceptions of ageing', *Preventative Medicine* 39:3, pp. 625-9.

16 Bratt, C., Abrams, D., Swift, H., Vauclair, C.M., and Marques, S. (2017), 'Perceived age discrimination across age in Europe: from an ageing society to a society for all ages', *Developmental Psychology* 54:1. pp. 167-180.

17 Stephan Y., Sutin A. and Terracciano A. (2015), 'How old do you feel? The role of age discrimination and biological aging in subjective age', *PLoS ONE* 10:3, pp.1-12.

18 Stephan, Y, Chalabaev, A., Kotter-Gruhn, D. and Jaconelli, A. (2013), 'Feeling younger, being stronger: an experimental study of subjective age and physical functioning among older adults', *Journals of Gerontology - Series B Psychological Sciences and Social Sciences* 68:1, pp. 1-7.

19 Preston, C., Drydakis, N., et al. (2018), *Planning and preparing for later life*, Centre for Ageing Better.

20 Hall, S., Rennick, K. and Williams, R. (2019), *The Perennials: The future of Ageing*, Ipsos MORI and Centre for Ageing Better.

21 Office for Budget Responsibility (2017), *Fiscal risks report.*

22 Willetts, D. (2019), p. 297.

23 Office of National Statistics, (2019), Annual Survey of Hours and Earnings data, 2018-based. Workplace analysis, income deciles of all full-time workers in the UK

24 Department for Work and Pensions (2011), *A sustainable State Pension: when the state pension age will increase to 66.*

25 Select Committee on Intergenerational Fairness and Provision (2019), *Tackling intergenerational unfairness, report of session 2017-19*, House of Lords.

26 Swales, K. (2016), *Understanding the Leave vote*, NatCen.

27 Calouste Gulbenkian and Royal Society for Public Health (2018), *That age old question: How attitudes to ageing affect our health and wellbeing*, Royal Society for Public Health.

28 Willetts, D. (2019), p. 293.

29 Intergenerational Commission (2018), *A new generational contract: The final report of the Intergenerational Commission*, Resolution Foundation.

30 Finch, D. and Rose, H. (2017), A mid-life less ordinary? Characteristics and incomes of low to middle income households aged 50 to State Pension age, Resolution Foundation and Centre for Ageing Better

31 Shrimpton, H., Skinner, G. and Hall, S. (2017), *The millennial bug: Public attitudes on the living standards of different generations*, Resolution Foundation, based on Ipsos Mori poll of 2,179 UK adults 16-75, May 2017.

CHAPTER 3 MONEY, MONEY, MONEY

1 Lloyd George, D. (1908), Hansard, Parliamentary Debates, House of Commons, 4th Series, vol. 140, Columns 565-586, June 1908.

2 Harris, J. (2006), *Pauper Progress: From Poor Relief to Old Age Pension*, National Pensioners Convention, Smallprint: London.

3 Office of National Statistics (2017), Period and cohort life expectancy explained.

4 Department for Work and Pensions (2019), *Households Below Average Income: An analysis of the UK income distribution: 1994/95-2017/18.*

5 Office of Budget Responsibility (2017), *Fiscal Sustainability Report.*

6 Department for Work and Pensions (2018), Income-related benefits: estimates of take-up: financial year 2016-17.

7 OECD (2017), *Pensions at a Glance: OECD and G20 Indicators*, OECD Publishing: Paris.

8 Pensions Policy Institute (2019), *The Pensions Primer: A guide to the UK pensions system.*

9 Johnson, P. (2013), 'Pensioner incomes in the UK', Institute for Fiscal Studies, Presentation to first CEPAR annual conference, 2 July 2013.

10 Pensions Policy Institute (2019)

11 Silcock, D., Pike, T. and Adams, J. (2018), *How would removal of the state pension triple lock affect adequacy?* Pensions Policy Institute.

12 Office of National Statistics (2018), Household disposable income and inequality, table 3a: Household characteristics of all households by decile group, 2016/17.

13 Joseph Rowntree Foundation (2019), based on estimated benefit take-up from calculated entitlement in the IPPR Tax-Benefit Model and reported receipt of the benefit in the Family Resources Survey.

14 Office for Budget Responsibility (2018), *Fiscal Sustainability Report*, July 2018.

15 Office of National Statistics (2015), *How has life expectancy changed over time?*

16 Office of National Statistics (2018), Health state life expectancy at birth and at age 65 by local areas, UK, 2015-2017-based.

17 Cridland, J. (2017), *Smoothing the transition, Independent Review of the State Pension Age*.

18 Department for Work and Pensions (2014), Fuller working lives: Background evidence base.

19 Bourquin, P., Cribb, J., Waters, T. and Xu, X. (2019), *Living standards, poverty and inequality in the UK*, Institute for Fiscal Studies.

20 DWP Tabulation Tool (2014), Great Britain: percentage of all claimants in receipt of the state pension, September 2014.

21 Turner, A., Drake, J. and Hills, J. (2005), *A new pension settlement for the twenty-first century: The second report of the Pensions Commission*, Department for Work and Pensions.

22 Older, C., Ripley, E., et al. (2017), *Understanding the financial lives of UK adults, Findings from the FCA's Financial Lives Survey 2017*, Financial Conduct Authority.

23 Department for Work and Pensions (2017), Pensioners' incomes series: financial year 2016/17.

24 McLeod, P., Fitzpatrick, A., et al. (2012), *Attitudes to pensions: The 2012 survey*, Department for Work and Pensions.

25 World Health Organization (2012), 'The health-care challenges posed by population ageing', *Bulletin of the World Health Organization* 90:2, pp.77-156.

26 International Monetary Fund (2019), *Brazil: Staff report for the 2019 Article IV Consultation*.

27 Brazilian Institute of Geography and Statistics, Brazil's Complete Table for Mortality 2013.

28 OECD (2017), *OECD policy memo: Pension reform in Brazil*.

29 HM Treasury (2018), Whole of government accounts, year ended 31 March 2017.

30 Franklin, B. and Hochlaf, D. (2017), *The global savings gap*, ILC-UK.

31 Office of National Statistics, Occupational pension schemes survey, table 12, 2017-based.

32 Department for Work and Pensions (2017), *Security and sustainability in defined benefit pension schemes*.

33 Bell, B. and Whittaker, M. (2017), *The pay deficit: Measuring the effect of pension deficit payments on workers' wages*, Intergenerational Commission and Resolution Foundation.

34 Legal and General (2018), *Annual Reports and Accounts 2018: Improving lives through inclusive capitalism*.

35 The Pensions Regulator (2017), Regulatory intervention report: issued under section 89 of the Pensions Act 2004 in relation to the BHS pension schemes.

36 Comptroller and Auditor General (2018), *Investigation into the government's handling of the collapse of Carillion*, National Audit Office/Cabinet Office.

37 Clery, E., Humphreys, A. and Bourne, T. (2010,) *Attitudes to pensions: The 2009 survey*, Department for Work and Pensions.

38 Department for Work and Pensions (2017), *Automatic Enrolment Review 2017: Maintaining the Momentum*.

39 IPSE (2018), *Exploring the rise of self-employment in the modern economy*.

40 Department for Work and Pensions (2019), Workplace pension participation and saving trends: 2008 to 2018.

41 Office of National Statistics, (2018), Occupational Pension Schemes Survey, 2017-based; Office of National Statistics, (2018), Estimates of the population for the UK, England and Wales, Scotland and Northern Ireland, mid-2017 based.

42 Ali, R., et al. (2011), Statistics on household wealth, Department for Work and Pensions, annuity estimate based on 65-year-old woman with defined contribution pensions worth a total of £20,000.

43 Silcock, D., Pike, T. and Adams, J. (2018)

44 Office of National Statistics (2018), Occupational Pension Schemes Survey.

45 Department for Work and Pensions (2017), *Automatic enrolment review 2017: Maintaining the momentum*.

46 Thaler, R. and Bernatzi, S. (2004), 'Save more tomorrow: Using behavioural economics to increase employee saving', *Journal of Political Economy* 112:1, pp. 164-187.

47 Sefton, T., Evandrou, M. and Falkingham, J. (2011), 'Family ties: Women's work and family histories and their association with incomes in later life in the UK', *Journal of Social Policy* 40:1, pp. 41-69.

48 Scharf, T. and Shaw, C. (2017), *Inequalities in later life: Scoping review*, Newcastle University Institute for Ageing, Institute of Health and Society and ILC-UK, commissioned by Centre for Ageing Better.

49 Johnson, P., Yeandle, D. and Boulding, A. (2010), *Making automatic enrolment work*, A review for the Department for Work and Pensions.

50 Department for Work and Pensions (2019), *Pensions dashboards: feasibility report and consultation*.

51 James, H. (2019), *Engagement pathways in workplace pensions*, Pensions Policy Institute.

52 Financial Conduct Authority (2018), *Retirement Outcomes Review*, analysis of Association of British Insurers data.

53 Financial Conduct Authority (2018), 'Findings from the FCA's Financial Lives survey', *Data Bulletin*, March 2018.

54 Financial Conduct Authority (2018), *Retirement Outcomes Review*, analysis of Association of British Insurers data.

55 Gratton, L. and Scott, A. (2016) *The 100-year life*, Bloomsbury: London.

56 Finch, D. (2017), *Live long and prosper? Demographic trends and their implications for living standards*, Intergenerational Commission.

57 Department for Work and Pensions (2019), *Delivering collective defined contribution pension schemes*, Consultation paper.

Chapter 4 The world of work

1 Jones, O. (2016), 'We should be striving to work less, not toiling until we drop', *Guardian*, 3 March 2016.

2 Perkins, A. (2015), 'The have-it-all generation has to be told when to quit', *Guardian*, 5 August 2015.

3 Office of National Statistics (2018), UK labour market: January 2018.

4 Annual Population Survey (2018), Labour market status by age, March 2018.

5 Aviva (2016), Aviva analysis of Labour Market Survey.

6 Chartered Institute of Personnel and Development (2015), *Avoiding the demographic crunch: Labour supply and the ageing workforce*, CIPD and ILC-UK.

7 Royal College of General Practitioners estimates, 2019 based.

8 Banks, J., Blundell, R., et al. (2008), *Releasing jobs for the young? Early retirement and youth unemployment in the UK*, IFS Working Paper W10/02, Institute for Fiscal Studies.

9 OECD. Stat, (2018), – Employment indicators, Labour Force Participation rate, 15-64 age group compared to 60-64, 2017-based.

10 Pacitti, C. and Smith, J. (2019), *A problem shared? What can we learn from past recessions about the impact of the next across the income distribution?* Resolution Foundation.

11 McNair, S., Worman, D. and Willmott, B. (2012), *Managing a healthy ageing workforce: A national business imperative*, Scottish Centre for Healthy Working Lives and Chartered Institute of Personnel and Development.

12 OECD (2017), Labour force participation rate, 65 years old or more, percentage in same age group.

13 OECD (2018), *Working better with age: Japan, ageing and employment policies*, OECD Publishing.

14 Japanese Institute for Labour Policy and Training, *Databook of International Labour Statistics 2017: Population and Labour Force*, 2015-based.

15 Kageyama, Y. (2018), 'Construction robots weld, bolt, lift to beat worker shortage', *AP News*, 23 April.

16 Ipsos MORI survey of 20,788 adults 16-64 in 30 countries, 24 August-7 September 2018.

17 Brown, T. (2017), Statistical profile of membership, House of Lords Library.

18 University of Oxford (2017), Employer Justified Retirement Age; University of Cambridge (2016), Retirement Policy.

19 Department for Work and Pensions, (2017), Fuller Working Lives Evidence Base: Annual Population Survey data, July 2015-June 2016.

20 Wainwright, D., Crawford, J., Loretto, W., et al. (2018), 'Extending working life and the management of change. Is the workplace ready for the ageing worker?', *Ageing and Society* 39:11, pp. 2397-2419.

21 ACAS (2011), *Age and the workplace: Putting the Equality Act 2010 and the removal of the default retirement age (DPA) into practice.*

22 Office of National Statistics, (2019), Annual Population Survey data 2010-2017, Employment rate by age group.

23 Ipsos Mori,(2015), *Later life in 2015: An analysis of the views and experiences of people aged 50 and over*, commissioned by the Centre for Ageing Better, sample of 1,389 adults over 50 in England.

24 Platts, L., Corna, L., et al. (2019), 'Returns to work after retirement: a prospective study of unretirement in the UK', *Ageing and Society* 39:3, pp 439-464.

25 NatCen, British Social Attitudes Survey (2008 and 2011).

26 Gessa, G., Corna, L., Price, D. and Glaser, K. (2018), 'The decision to work after state pension age and how it affects quality of life: evidence from a 6-year English panel study', *Age and Ageing* 47:3, pp. 1-8.

27 Topping, A. (2016), 'Eager 89-year-old seeks job: cafe snaps him up', *Guardian*, 1 December 2016.

28 Marvell, R. and Cox, A. (2017), *What do older workers value about work and why?*, Institute for Employment Studies and Centre for Ageing Better.

29 Centre for Ageing Better (2017), IFF survey of 500 employers, Poll shows UK employers unprepared for managing ageing workforce, October 2017.

30 Department for Work and Pensions (2016), *Attitudes to working in later life: British social attitudes in 2016*.

31 Timewise Flexible Jobs Index 2018.

32 Marvell, R. and Cox, A. (2017), *What do older workers value about work and why?*, Institute for Employment Studies and Centre for Ageing Better.

33 YouGov (2018), *Becoming an age-friendly employer*, commissioned by Centre for Ageing Better.

34 Drydakis, N., MacDonald, P., Chiotis, V. and Somers, L. (2017), 'Age discrimination in the UK labour market: Does race moderate ageism? An experimental investigation', *Applied Economics Letters* 25:1, pp. 1-4.

35 Ofcom (2018), *Diversity and equal opportunities in television: Monitoring report on the UK-based broadcasting industry*.

36 Recruitment and Employment Confederation and Age UK (2015), *Age Opportunity: A best practice guide for recruiters*.

37 Abrams, D., Swift, H. and Drury, L. (2016), 'Old and unemployable? How age-based stereotypes affect willingness to hire job candidates', *Journal of Social Issues* 72:1, pp.105-121.

38 Schmiedek, F., Loevden, M. and Lindenberger, U (2010), 'Hundred days of cognitive training enhance broad cognitive abilities in adulthood: findings from the COGITO study', *Frontiers in Aging Neuroscience* 2:27.

39 HM Government (2015) *Supporting working carers: The benefits to families, businesses* and the economy, Final report of the Carers in Employment Task and Finish group, Carers UK and Employers for Carers.

40 Centrica, (2015), Best for Carers and Eldercare, Top Employers for Working Families Special Awards 2015, Centrica estimate.

41 YouGov and Mustard Research (2018), *Health warning for employers: Supporting older workers with health conditions*, for Centre for Ageing Better.

42 Loch, C.H., Sting, F., Bauer N. and Mauermann, H. (2010), 'How BMW Is defusing the demographic time bomb', *Harvard Business Review* 88:3, pp. 99-102.

43 Centre for Ageing Better and Calouste Gulbenkian Foundation (2017), Evaluation of Transitions in Later Life pilot projects.

44 OECD (2012), *Education at a Glance: Highlights*, OECD Publishing.

45 Gratton, L. and Scott, A. (2016), *The 100-year Life*, Bloomsbury: London.

46 Centre for Ageing Better (2018), *Developing the mid-life MOT*.

47 Chartered Institute of Personnel and Development (2014), *Managing an age-diverse workforce: Employer and employee views*.

48 Department for Work and Pensions, DWP equality information 2016: employee data, data table 6 (performance) and 7 (promotion).

49 Marvell R. and Cox, A. (2017), *What do older workers value about work and why?*, Institute for Employment Studies and Centre for Ageing Better.

50 Mercer (2019), *Next age, next stage: A new approach to aging and longevity*.

51 Department of Business, Energy and Industrial Strategy (2017), *Industrial Strategy: Building a Britain fit for the future*.

52 Department of Business, Energy and Industrial Strategy (2018), *Business Productivity Review: Government call for evidence*.

53 Office of National Statistics, (2019), Annual Population Survey data: Labour market status by age, July 2018 to June 2019.

54 Office of National Statistics (2017), Economic activity of people with disabilities defined under the Equality Act 2010, October 2015-September 2016, England and Wales, user requested data, reference no. 006735, 2015-2016-based.

55 HM Treasury (2018), *Managing fiscal risks: Government response to the 2017 fiscal risks report*.

56 Office of National Statistics, (2017), Annual Population Survey data: Economic activity by single year of age, July 2015-June 2016.

57 Office of National Statistics, Labour Force Survey A01: Summary of labour market statistics, Table 2: Labour market activity by age group (seasonally adjusted), February-April 2019.

58 Office of National Statistics (2018), Health state life expectancy at birth and at age 65 by local areas, UK.

59 Franklin, B. et al. (2014), *The Missing million: Illuminating the employment challenges of the over-50s*, Business in the Community.

60 Department for Work and Pensions (2018), Employment and Support Allowance caseload, Stat Xplore, February 2018.

61 Health and Safety Executive (2018), Workplace fatal injuries in Great Britain.

62 Health and Safety Executive (2017), *Historical picture – trends in work-related ill health and workplace injury in Great Britain.*

63 Health and Safety Executive (2018), Work-related stress, depression or anxiety statistics in Great Britain.

64 Mayhew, L. (2018), *The Dependency Trap – are we fit enough to face the future?*, University of London: Centre for the Study of Financial Innovation.

65 Banks, J., Batty, G.D., et al. (2016), *The dynamics of ageing: Evidence from the English Longitudinal Study of Ageing, Wave 8: 2002-2015*, Institute for Fiscal Studies.

66 NHS (2019), The NHS Long Term Plan.

67 Office of National Statistics (2019), Unemployment by age and duration (seasonally adjusted), February-April 2019.

68 Department for Work and Pensions (2014), Fuller working lives - Background evidence.

69 Department for Work and Pensions (2018), Work programme statistical summary: data to December 2017.

70 Age UK (2016), *Helping 50+ jobseekers back to work: lessons for the Work and Health Programme.*

71 Centre for Ageing Better (2017), *Addressing worklessness and job insecurity among people aged 50 and over in Greater Manchester.*

72 Chandola, T. and Zhang, N. (2017), 'Re-employment, job quality, health and allostatic load biomarkers: prospective evidence from the UK Household Longitudinal Study', *International Journal of Epidemiology* 47:1, pp. 47-57.

73 Irvine, G., White, D. and Diffley, D. (2018), *Measuring good work: The final report of the Measuring Job Quality Working Group*, Carnegie UK and RSA.

74 What Works Wellbeing (2017), What is a good job? Analysis based on findings from the British 2012 Skills and Employment Survey.

75 Wallace-Stephens, F. (2019), *Economic insecurity: The case for a 21st century safety net*, Royal Society of Arts, Manufactures and Commerce, and Center for Inclusive Growth.

76 AirBnB (2016), Senior hosts fastest growing demographic in Europe.

77 McKay, S. and Simpson, I. (2015), *Work: Attitudes and experiences of work in a changing labour market*, British Attitudes Survey.

78 Association of Independent Professionals and the Self-Employed (2017), *Exploring the rise of self-employment in the modern economy: A guide to demographics and other trends in the UK's self-employed workforce in 2017*, analysis of Labour Force Survey.

79 Office of National Statistics (2018), *Trends in self-employment in the UK*.

80 Department for Business, Energy and Industrial Strategy (2018), *The characteristics of those in the gig economy*.

81 Department for Business, Energy and Industrial Strategy (2019), *Good work plan: Consultation on measures to address one-sided flexibility*.

CHAPTER 5 WHAT WE DO WITH OUR TIME

1 Booth, C. (1898), Address to old age pension campaign conference, Browning Hall.

2 Gratton, L. and Scott, L. (2016), *The 100-Year Life*, Bloomsbury: London.

3 Garcia, H. and Mirrales, F. (2016), *Ikigai: The Japanese Secret to a Long and Happy Life*, trans. Heather Cleary, Hutchinson: London.

4 Office of National Statistics (2018), Personal wellbeing in the UK: January to December 2017.

5 YouGov (2017), *Retirement transitions in later life*, commissioned by Centre for Ageing Better and Calouste Gulbenkian Foundation.

6 Abell J., Amin-Smith, N., et al. (2018), *The dynamics of ageing: Evidence from the English Longitudinal Study of Ageing, Wave 8: 2002-2016*, Institute for Fiscal Studies.

7 Jagger, C., Gillies, C., et al. (2008) 'Inequalities in healthy life years in the 25 countries of the European Union in 2005: a cross-national meta-regression analysis', *The Lancet* 372, pp. 2124-213.

8 Barnes, H. and Parry, J. (2004), 'Renegotiating identity and relationships: men and women's adjustments to retirement', *Ageing and Society* 24:2, pp. 213-233.

9 Preston, C., Drydakis, N., et al. (2018), *Planning and preparing for later life*, Anglia Ruskin University and Centre for Ageing Better.

10 Centre for Ageing Better and Calouste Gulbenkian Foundation (2017*), Evaluation of transitions in Later Life pilot projects*.

11   Evans, E., Hyde, M., Davies, J., Moffatt, S., O'Brien, N and Windle G. (2019), Navigating later life transitions: An evaluation of emotional and psychological interventions, Calouste Gulbenkian Foundation and Centre for Ageing Better.

12   NCVO (2018), Volunteering participation estimates based on the Community Life Survey, 2017-18.

13   Kamarade, D. (2011), 'An untapped pool of volunteers for the Big Society? Not enough social capital? Depends on how you measure it', in *Voluntary Sector Studies Network Day Conference*, Cardiff University.

14   Department for Digital, Culture and Media (2019), Community Life Survey 2018-19.

15   Mohan, J. and Bulloch, S. (2012), *The idea of a 'civic core': what are the overlaps between charitable giving, volunteering, and civic participation in England and Wales?*, Third Sector Research Centre.

16   Nazroo, J. and Matthews, K. (2012), *The impact of volunteering on wellbeing in later life*, London: (WRVS) Royal Voluntary Services.

17   Jones, D. and Jopling, K. (2018), *Age-friendly and inclusive volunteering: Review of community contributions in later life*, Centre for Ageing Better.

18   Department of Culture, Media and Sport, Community Life Survey, 2012-2017.

19   Centre for Ageing Better (2018), Primary research into community contributions in later life.

20   Jones, D., Young A. and Reeder, N. (2016), *The benefits of making a contribution to your community in later life*, Evidence briefing, Centre for Ageing Better.

21   Nazroo, J. and Matthews, K. (2012)

22   Kamerade, D and Paine, A. (2014), 'Volunteering and employability: implications for policy and practice', *Voluntary Sector Review* 5:2, pp. 259-73.

23   Iparraguirre, J. (2018), *The economic contribution of older people in the United Kingdom: An update to 2017*, Age UK.

24   NCVO (2019), Time Well Spent Survey: survey of more than 10,000 UK adults over 16.

25   Nazroo, J.Y. (2015) *Volunteering, providing informal care and paid employment in later life: Role occupancy and implications for wellbeing*, Future of ageing: Evidence review, Foresight, Government Office for Science.

26 Van der Horst, M., Vickerstaff, S., Lain, D., Clark, C., Baumberg Geiger, B. (2017), 'Pathways of paid work, care provision and volunteering in later careers: Activity substitution or extension?', *Work, Aging & Retirement* 3:4, pp. 343-365.

27 Nazroo, J.Y. (2015)

28 Lancee, B. and Radl, J. (2014), 'Volunteering over the life course', *Social Forces* 93:2, pp. 833-862.

29 Rochester, C., Paine, A.E., et al. (2010), *Volunteering and Society in the 21st Century*, Palgrave Macmillan.

30 Office of National Statistics, 2011, Census data – Provision of unpaid care – all.

31 NHS Digital (2019), Personal social services survey of adult carers in England, 2018-19.

32 Office of National Statistics, 2011, Census data – Provision of unpaid care – by age.

33 Pickard, L. (2012), 'Substitution between formal and informal care: a 'natural experiment' in social policy in Britain between 1985 and 2000', *Ageing and Society* 32: 7, pp. 1147-75.

34 Pickard, L. (2015), 'A growing care gap? The supply of unpaid care for older people by their adult children in England to 2032', *Ageing and Society* 35:1, pp. 96-123.

CHAPTER 6 HEALTHY, LONGER LIVES – IS IT ALL DOWNHILL FROM HERE?

1 Peev, G. (2013), 'An ageing population has pushed the NHS and social care system to the brink of collapse, the health minister Norman Lamb has warned...', *Daily Mail*, 13th May 2013.

2 Office of Budget Responsibility (2018), *Fiscal Sustainability Report*.

3 Evans, R., quoted in Beckett, C. and Maynard, A. (2005), *Value and Ethics in Social Work*, Sage: London.

4 Office of National Statistics (2019), Gross Domestic Product: Year on Year growth: CVM SA %, average between 1978 and 2018.

5 Seshamani, M. and Gray, A. (2004), 'Time to death and health expenditure: an improved model for the impact of demographic change on health care costs', *Ageing and Society* 33:6, pp. 556-561.

6 Bardsley, M., Georghiou, T. and Dixon, J. (2010), *Social care and hospital use at the end of life*, Nuffield Trust.

7   Cooper, MH, and Culyer, A.J. (1967), An economic assessment of some aspects of the Operation of the National Health Service, in Jones, I.M. (ed), *Health Service Financing*, British Medical Association.

8   Gawande, A. (2014), *Being Mortal: Medicine and What Matters in the End*, New York: Macmillan.

9   Resuscitation Council (2014), Decisions about Cardiopulmonary Resuscitation (CPR).

10 Connor, S., Pyenson, B., et al. (2007), 'Comparing hospice and nonhospice patient survival among patients who die within a three-year window', *Journal of Pain and Symptom Management* 33:3, pp. 238-246.

11 Temel, J., Greer, J., et al. (2010), 'Early palliative care for patients with metastatic non–small-cell lung cancer', *New England Journal of Medicine* 363:8, pp. 733-742.

12 Lloyd, T., Walters, A. and Stevenson, A. (2017), *The impact of providing enhanced support for care home residents in Rushcliffe: consideration of findings from the Improvement Analytics Unit*, The Health Foundation.

13 Forder, J. and Fernandez, J-L. (2011), *Length of stay in care homes*, report commissioned by Bupa Care Services, PSSRU Discussion Paper 2769, Personal Social Services Research Unit.

14 NatCen survey for Dying Matters of 1,375 people over 16 in England, Scotland and Wales, July-September 2009.

15 Omran, AR (1971), 'The epidemiologic transition: A theory of the epidemiology of population change', *The Milbank Memorial Fund Quarterly*, 49:4, pp. 509-38.

16 Cooper, MH, and Culyer, AJ (1967)

17 Melzer, D., Tavakoly, B., Winder, R., Richards, S., Gericke, C. and Lang, I. (2012), *Health care quality for an active later life: Improving quality of prevention and treatment through information – England 2005 to 2012*, Peninsula College of Medicine and Dentistry Ageing Research Group for Age UK, University of Exeter.

18 Department for Work and Pensions, (2017), Fuller Working Lives Evidence Base: Annual Population Survey data, July 2015-July 2016.

19 Office of National Statistics, Health state life expectancy – all ages, UK, 2015-2017-based.

20 Office of National Statistics (2015), Trend in life expectancy at birth and at age 65 by socio-economic position based on the

National Statistics socio-economic classification, England and Wales: 1982-1986 to 2007-2011.

21 Office of National Statistics, Health state life expectancies by national deprivation deciles, England and Wales: 2015 to 2017.

22 Marmot, M. (2010), *Fair Society, Healthy Lives: The Marmot Review*, Institute of Health Equity.

23 Pickett, R. and Wilkinson, K. (2015), *The Spirit Level: Why More Equal Societies Almost Always Do Better*, Allen Lane, London.

24 Nazroo, J. (2017), Class and health inequality in later life: Patterns, mechanisms and implications for policy, *International Journal of Environmental Research and Public Health*, 14:2.

25 Stoye, G. (2017), *UK health spending*, Institute for Fiscal Studies and Nuffield Foundation.

26 Institute for Health Metrics and Evaluation (2018), Global Burden of Disease Study, UK Profile.

27 Rissel, C., Curac, N., et al. (2012), 'Physical activity associated with public transport use—a review and modelling of potential benefits', *International Journal of Environmental Research and Public Health* 9:7, pp. 454-2478.

28 Thaler, R. and Sunstein, C. (2009), *Nudge: Improving Decisions About Health, Wealth and Happiness*, Penguin: New York.

29 Marteau, T., et al. (2019), 'Increasing healthy life expectancy equitably in England by 5 years by 2035: could it be achieved?', comment piece, *The Lancet*, 393:10191, pp. 2571-2573.

30 Office of National Statistics (2018), Adult smoking habits in England.

31 NHS Digital (2019), Health Survey for England, 2012-2018.

32 Royal College of Psychiatrists (2018), *Our invisible addicts*, 2nd edition.

33 Office of National Statistics, Adult Drinking Habits in England, 2017 data.

34 NHS Digital (2018), Statistics on alcohol, England-2018

35 Drinkwise Age Well, Where we work.

36 NHS Digital (2018), Statistics on obesity, physical activity and diet – England.

37 Wang, Y.C., et al. (2011), 'Health and economic burden of the projected obesity trends in the USA and the UK', *The Lancet* 378, pp. 815-825.

38 World Health Organisation (2017), Taxes on sugary drinks: why do it?

39 Health Survey for England (2012), Health, social care and lifestyles.

40 Campbell, F., Holmes, M., Everson-Hock, E., Davis, S., Woods, H.B., Anokye, N., et al (2015), 'A systematic review and economic evaluation of exercise referral schemes in primary care: a short report', *Health Technology Assessment* 19(60).

41 Office of National Statistics, Measuring national wellbeing: Quality of life in the UK, 2016-based data.

42 NHS Digital (2005), Health Survey for England – Health of older people.

43 Burns, A. (2015), 'Better access to mental health services for older people', NHS England blog.

44 Centre for Ageing Better and Calouste Gulbenkian Foundation (2017), *Evaluation of transitions in Later Life pilot projects*.

45 Blackburn, E. and Espel, E. (2017), *The Telomere Effect: A revolutionary approach to living younger, healthier, longer*, Grand Central Publishing: New York.

46 McCartney, M. (2012), 'Would you like your telomeres tested?', *BMJ*, comment piece.

47 World Health Organisation (2018), *International Classification of Diseases*, 11th edition, MG2A: Old Age.

CHAPTER 7 WHO CARES?

1 Anonymous social worker, (2019), 'It's time to declare a social care emergency', 21st August 2019, *Guardian*

2 Griffiths, D., et al. (2018), *The state of the adult social care sector and workforce in England*, Skills for Care.

3 Franklin, B. (2014), *The future care workforce*, ILC-UK.

4 The Health Foundation, Nuffield Trust and the King's Fund (2017), Autumn Budget: Joint statement on health and social care.

5 Local Government Association (2018), *The lives we want to lead: Findings, implications and recommendations on the LGA green paper for adult social care and wellbeing*, consultation response.

6 Institute of Public Care (2017), *Market shaping in adult social care*, Oxford Brookes University.

7 Lievesley, N., Cooper, G. and Bowman, C. (2011), *The changing role of care homes*, Centre for Policy on Ageing and Bupa.

8 Jefferson, L., Bennett, L., et al. (2018), *Home care in England: Views from commissioners and providers*, The King's Fund.

9   HMRC (2013), National Minimum Wage compliance in the social care sector: An evaluation of National Minimum Wage enforcement in the social care sector over the period 1 April 2011 to 31 March 2013.

10 Bottery, S. (2018), *Home care in England: Views from commissioners and providers*, King's Fund: London.

11 LaingBuisson (2018), *Care of older people UK market report*, 29th edition.

12 National Audit Office (2018), *Adult social care at a glance*.

13 Care Quality Commission, *The state of health care and adult social care in England, 2017-18*.

14 Office of National Statistics, 2011 Census data – Provision of unpaid care – all.

15 Pickard, L. (2015), 'A growing care gap? The supply of unpaid care for older people by their adult children in England to 2032', *Ageing and Society* 35:1, pp. 96-123.

16 Brimblecombe, N., et al (2018), *Unpaid Care in England: Future Patterns and Potential Support Strategies*, Personal Social Services Research Unit: London.

17 Office of National Statistics (2019), *Living longer: caring in later working life*.

18 Curry, N., Schlepper, L and Hemmings, N. (2019), *What can England learn from the long-term care system in Germany?*, Nuffield Trust.

19 Destatis, Statistisches Bundesamt (2017), Die Kinderlosigkeit in Deutschland ist nicht weiter gestiegen.

20 Office of National Statistics (2018), Childbearing for women born in different years.

21 Centre for Policy on Ageing (2016), Foresight future of an ageing population – International case studies, case study 8: Long term care insurance in Germany.

22 National Audit Office (2017), Investigation into NHS continuing health care funding, Department of Health and NHS England.

23 Alders, P. and Schut, F. (2019), 'The 2015 long-term care reform in the Netherlands: Getting the financial incentives right?', *Health Policy* 123:3, pp. 312-316.

24 NHS (2018) Health Survey for England – Adult social care.

25 Department for Work and Pensions (2018), Family Resources Survey 2016/17.

26 Kingston, A., et al. (2017), 'Is late-life dependency increasing or not? A comparison of the cognitive function and ageing studies (CFAS)', *The Lancet* 390:10103, pp. 1676-1684.

27 Kent integrated dataset, Mean annual cost of care by frailty category, KID population aged 65+, Jan-Dec 2017.

28 Office of National Statistics (2018), Health state life expectancies: 2014 to 2016.

29 Public Health England (2018), *Falls: applying All Our Health*, guidance.

30 Department of Health and Social Care (2019), UK Chief Medical Officers' Physical Activity Guidelines.

31 Grimby, G. and Saltin, B. (1983), 'The ageing muscle', *Clinical Physiology* 3:3, pp.209-218.

32 National Hip Fracture Database (2016), Annual Report 2016, Royal College of Physicians.

33 McNally, S., Nunan, D., Dixon, A., Maruthappu, M., Butler, K. and Gray, M. (2017), 'Focus on physical activity can help avoid unnecessary social care', *BMJ 359*.

34 Public Health England and the Centre for Ageing Better (2018), *Muscle and bone strengthening and balance activities for general health benefits in adults and older adults*, Summary of a rapid evidence review for the UK Chief Medical Officers' update of the physical activity guidelines.

35 Department of Health and Social Care (2019), *UK Chief Medical Officers' Physical Activity Guidelines.*

36 Centre for Ageing Better (2019), *Raising the bar on strength and balance: The importance of community-based provision.*

37 Oomph (2018), *The Oomph Impact Report 2017/18.*

38 NHS England (2018), *Quick guide: Technology in care homes.*

39 Department of Health and Social Care (2011), Whole system demonstrator evaluation.

40 Abdi, J., Al-Hindawi, A., et al. (2018), 'Scoping review on the use of socially assistive robot technology in elderly care', *BMJ Open*, 8:2.

CHAPTER 8 HOME SWEET HOME – OR IS IT?

1 Ipsos MORI (2016), Tenure and social mobility: Survey findings.

2 Ministry of Housing, Communities and Local Government (2019), English Housing Survey 2017-2018.

3   Bangham, G. (2019), *Game of homes: The rise of multiple property ownership in Great Britain*, Analysis of wealth and assets survey, Resolution Foundation.

4   Gardiner, L. (2017), *The million dollar be-question: Inheritances, gifts and their implications for generational living standards*, Resolution Foundation Intergenerational Commission.

5   Legal and General (2018), *Bank of Mum and Dad.*

6   Price Waterhouse Cooper (2016), *Housing market outlook*, UK Economic Outlook.

7   Gardiner, L. (2017)

8   Department for Communities and Local Government (2014), English Housing Survey 2014-2015.

9   Hammond, M., White, S. and Walsh, S. (2018), *Rightsizing: Reframing the housing offer for older people*, Manchester School of Architecture supported by the Centre for Ageing Better.

10 Burgess, G., Jones, M. and Muir, K. (2017), *Moving insights from the over-55s: What homes do they buy?*, National House-Buying Council.

11 Hammond, M., White, S. and Walsh, S. (2018)

12 National Audit Office (2019), Help to buy: Equity loan scheme – progress review, Ministry of Housing, Communities and Local Government.

13 Office of National Statistics (2019), Housing affordability in England and Wales: 2018.

14 Office of National Statistics (2014), Families and households in the UK: 2014.

15 Ministry of Housing, Communities and Local Government (2014), Live tables on dwelling stock (including vacants).

16 Ministry of Housing, Communities and Local Government (2019), Live tables on house building: new build dwellings, Permanent dwellings completed by tenure, 2000-2018.

17 Davis, B., et. al (2016), *German model homes? A comparison of UK and German housing markets*, Institute for Public Policy Research.

18 Ministry of Housing, Communities and Local Government (2014), Live tables on dwelling stock (including vacants).

19 Office of Budget Responsibility (2018), *Economic and fiscal outlook: October 2018.*

20 Pannell, J., Aldridge, H. and Kenway, P. (2012), *Market assessment of housing options for older people: A report for Shelter and the Joseph Rowntree Foundation*, New Policy Institute.

21 Department for Communities and Local Government (2018), 2016-based household projections: England, 2016-2041.

22 Hammond, M., White, S. and Walsh, S. (2018), (data from British Household Panel Survey and Understanding Society Survey, 1991-2017).

23 Department for Communities and Local Government (2014), Housing Standards Review, Cost Impacts.

24 Mackintosh, S. and Leather, P. (2016), *The Disabled Facilities Grant: Before and after the introduction of the Better Care Fund*, Foundations.

25 Ministry of Housing, Communities and Local Government (2018), English Housing Survey 2017-2018.

26 Lloyd, J. (2015), 'Older Owners Research on the lives, aspirations and housing outcomes of older homeowners in the UK', London: Strategic Society Centre.

27 Nicol, S., Roys, M., Ormandy, D. and Ezratty, V. (2016), *The cost of poor housing in the European Union*, BRE Press Briefing Paper.

28 Department of Community and Local Government (2006), *A decent home: definition and guidance for implementation*.

29 Department for Communities and Local Government (2014), English Housing Survey 2014-2015.

30 Garrett, H. and Burris, S. (2015), *Homes and ageing in England*, BRE Bracknell, IHS BRE Press.

31 Building Research Establishment (2011), *The cost of poor housing to the NHS*.

32 Hackett, P. (2019), *The hidden costs of poor-quality housing in the North*, A discussion paper for the Northern Housing Consortium, Smith Institute.

33 Leather, P., Nevin, B., Cole, I and Eadson, W. (2012), *The Housing Market Renewal Programme in England: development, impact and legacy*, Centre for Regional, Economic and Social Research, Sheffield Hallam University.

34 Department of Communities and Local Government (2016) *English Housing Survey, Adaptations and Accessibility Report, 2014-2015*.

35 Centre for Ageing Better (2017), *Room to improve: The role of home adaptations in improving later life*.

36 Bailey, C. and Hodgson, P. (2018), Primary research with practitioners and people with lived experience – to understand

the role of home adaptations in improving later life, Northumbria University and the Centre for Ageing Better.

37 Adams, S. and Hodges, M. (2018), *Adapting for ageing: Good practice and innovation in home adaptations*, Care and Repair England and Centre for Ageing Better.

38 Ministry of Housing, Communities and Local Government (2019), *English Housing Survey 2017-2018*.

39 All-Party Parliamentary Group: Housing and Care for Older People (2019) *Rental Housing for an Ageing Population*.

40 Department for Work and Pensions (2018), Benefit expenditure and caseload tables 2018, Outturn and Forecast: Autumn Budget 2018.

41 Clarke, S. (2018), *The future fiscal cost of 'Generation Rent'*, Resolution Foundation Intergenerational Centre.

42 Evandrou, M., Falkingham, J. and Green, M. (2010), 'Migration in later life: evidence from the British Household Panel Study', *Population Trends* 141 pp. 77-94.

43 Shelter (2016), *Green Book: 50 Years On, The reality of homelessness for families today*.

44 Mackintosh, S. and Leather, P. (2016), *The Disabled Facilities Grant: Before and after the introduction of the Better Care Fund*, Foundations.

45 Ministry of Housing, Communities and Local Government (2019), English Housing Survey 2017-2018.

46 Ministry of Housing, Communities and Local Government (2019), Live tables on affordable housing supply.

CHAPTER 9 THE LONELINESS MYTH AND WHY THE PLACE
WE LIVE MATTERS

1 Department for Digital, Culture, Media and Sport (2018), Community Life Survey 2017-18.

2 Jopling, K. (2017), *Combatting loneliness one conversation at a time: A call to action*, Jo Cox Loneliness Commission.

3 Smith, K. and Victor, C. (2019), 'Typologies of loneliness, living alone and social isolation, and their associations with physical and mental health', *Ageing and Society* 39:8, pp. 1709-1730.

4 Durcan, D. and Bell, R. (2015), *Reducing social isolation across the life course*, Public Health England and UCL Institute of Health Equity.

5 Centre for Ageing Better Analysis (2018), Understanding Society: The UK Household Longitudinal Study, Wave 6, 2014-16.

6 Scharf, T. and Shaw, C. (2017), *Inequalities in later life: scoping review*, Centre for Ageing Better.

7 Iparraguirre, J. (2018), *The economic contribution of older people in the United Kingdom: An update to 2017*, Age UK.

8 Beth Johnson Foundation (2016), *Our Voices: The experiences of people ageing without children.*

9 Murray, R. (2016), *The Living Well impact: A stock take of what we know so far*, NHS Kernow.

10 Victor, C. (2018), *An overview of reviews: the effectiveness of interventions to address loneliness at all stages of the life course*, What Works Centre for Wellbeing.

11 Fried, L., et al. (2013), 'Experience Corps: A dual trial to promote the health of older adults and children's academic success', *Contemporary Clinical Trials* 36(1), pp. 1-13.

12 Garcia, H. and Miralles, F. (2017), *Ikigai: the Japanese secret to a long and happy life*, Hutchinson.

13 Department for Digital, Culture, Media and Sport (2019), Community Life Survey 2013/14 and 2017/18.

14 Cuomo. A. (2018), 'New York: First Age-Friendly State in the Nation', *AARP International: The Journal*, vol. 11, pp. 24-27.

15 Centre for Ageing Better (2019), Ageing and mobility: A grand challenge.

16 Deloitte (2016*), There's no place like phone: Consumer usage patterns in the era of peak smartphone*, Global Mobile Consumer Survey.

17 Keles, B., McCrae, N. and Grealish, A. (2019), 'A systematic review: the influence of social media on depression, anxiety and psychological distress in adolescents', *International Journal of Adolescence and Youth*.

18 Victor, C. (2018), *An overview of reviews: the effectiveness of interventions to address loneliness at all stages of the life course*, What Works Centre for Wellbeing.

19 Richardson, J. (2018), *I am connected: New approaches to supporting people in later life online*, Good Things Foundation and Centre for Ageing Better.

Acknowledgements

The seeds of this book were planted when the Centre for Ageing Better was still a start-up. Louise Ansari, Director of Communications, and Charlotte Croft from Bloomsbury, who was later to become my editor, came up with the crazy idea to publish a book. At the time I did not have much to write about. Today, the Centre for Ageing Better is a well-established and highly-regarded organisation that has gathered a wealth of knowledge about the changes needed in society so everyone can enjoy later life.

I am indebted to all the staff at the Centre for Ageing Better on whose work much of this book rests and without whom it could not have been written; to those colleagues, particularly Louise Ansari, who read early versions and provided helpful suggestions; and above all to Amy McSweeney who provided invaluable research support, was tireless in her pursuit of sources and references, checking facts and statistics, and responding to a deluge of questions and queries.

I have learnt so much over the past four years since taking on my role as Chief Executive at the Centre for Ageing Better. Many people have influenced my thinking and the ideas which are set out in this book. There are too many people to acknowledge individually; I am grateful for the interactions I have had with expert academics, leading practitioners and business leaders, senior policymakers, my peers in other ageing organisations, colleagues in the third sector, and the people I have met at North London Cares and other local groups who have shared their personal stories with me.

Many of these people have been working on these issues for longer than I have and yet have been willing to share their knowledge, wisdom and experiences with me. I am particularly grateful to the following people who generously gave their time to share their insights and expertise:

Muir Gray
Julia Randell-Khan
Phillip Brown
John Beard
John Cridland
Jeremy Porteus
Matthew Taylor
Zoe Wyrko
Kalpa Kharicha
Andy Briggs
Christina Victor

I would also like to thank the individuals and organisations whose work contributed to the case studies and helped source material for the book including the Calouste Gulbenkian Foundation, Natasha Curry at the Nuffield Trust, Dawn Newsome at Armley Helping Hands, Mary Bright and colleagues at Aviva, Laura Gardiner at the Resolution Foundation, and John Adams and Daniela Silcock at Pensions Policy Institute.

I could not have written this book alongside being a Chief Executive without the support of my current and past Chairs, Lord Filkin and Dame Carol Black, my wonderful colleagues who supported me to have days working from home to write, my husband David for being there through it all and tolerating the laptop coming on holiday, my friends who believed I could, my parents who welcomed me back 'home' to lock myself away in the attic and get the final manuscript written, and the positive encouragement of my editor Charlotte Croft.

The views and opinions in this book are mine and not those of the Centre for Ageing Better and I take full responsibility for any errors of commission or omission.

Index

Page numbers in italics are figures.